PHARMACEUTICAL PHD THESIS WRITING AND CONDUCTING THE RESEARCH STEP-BY-STEP GUIDANCE

Topic Selection to Submission. All streams and Branches!

PATHAN AZHER KHAN

M.PHARMACY, PhD

PAYAL JAYENDRA BADOLE

Scientific Researcher

SWARUPA MOHAN WANOLE

Scientific Writer

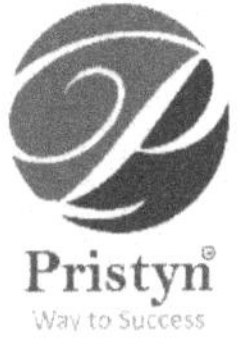

Pristyn®
Way to Success

Published by: Pristyn Research Solutions ®

*"Formal education will make you a living;
self-education will make you a fortune."
- Jim Rohn.*

Edition; 2024.

Published By: Pristyn Research Solutions ®
Plot No. T-21/4, Software Technology Park of India (STPI),
Next to Devgiri Software, Chikalthana MIDC, Aurangabad,
Maharashtra-431006, INDIA.
Phone: 09028839789 | 9028912522
e-Mail: info@pristynresearch.com | Website: www.pristynresearch.com

Note: Despite ongoing efforts for accuracy, new information may
necessitate changes. Neither editors nor publishers can guarantee
completeness due to human error or scientific progress.

Table of Content

Chapter 1

TOPIC SELECTION STRATEGIES

Select a topic that fuels your passion,

1.1 What is a pharmaceutical PhD?

An advanced research degree with a pharmaceutical sciences concentration is called a PhD in pharmaceutical sciences, or a Doctor of Philosophy in Pharmaceutical Sciences. It entails in-depth investigation and analysis of numerous facets of medication delivery, development, discovery, and use. Choosing to pursue a PhD in pharmaceuticals has many benefits. First, it enables people to delve deeply into pharmaceutical research subfields, offering insightful new perspectives to the discipline. Second, PhD candidates can obtain some crucial advantages by doing extensive investigation and experimentation:

- Addresses pressing societal issues such as healthcare access, environmental sustainability, poverty alleviation, and technological innovation.
- Patent approval and protect intellectual property.
- Pharmaceutical research and innovation attract collaborations and partnerships with international organizations, academic institutions, and industry players.
- Develop advanced analytical and problem-solving skills that are essential for tackling complex industry challenges and advancing scientific knowledge (1).
- Personal growth and development of specific skills to become an expert.
- Improved communication skills while sharing knowledge.

A PhD program in pharmaceuticals usually lasts three to six years, depending on variables like the type of research, program requirements, individual advancement, etc. This period covers coursework, research projects, and thesis preparation, guaranteeing in-depth instruction and in-depth subject investigation.(2). Several fundamental fields of pharmacy provide a variety of opportunities for research and development. These consist of, but are not restricted to:

a) **Pharmacology**: The investigation of possible therapeutic uses, the comprehension of pharmacological mechanisms of action, and the research of how pharmaceuticals affect biological systems (3).

b) **Pharmaceutics:** This field is concerned with the formulation, manufacture, evaluation, and distribution of pharmacological dosage forms to maximize therapeutic efficacy and patient outcomes.

c) **Pharmaceutical chemistry:** Investigating the creation, synthesis, and characterisation of new pharmaceutical substances with enhanced pharmacological qualities.

d) **Pharmacokinetics and Pharmacodynamics:** Studying how medications interact with biological targets and are absorbed, distributed, metabolized, excreted, and toxic (ADMET) in the body (4,5).

e) **Clinical pharmacy**: Evaluating the safe and effective use of medications in patient care settings, emphasizing personalized treatment approaches and medication management.

f) **Pharmacognosy**: Investigate the identification of novel bioactive substances or natural sources derived from herbal remedies, look into their modes of action, and create novel therapeutic agents (6).

These core branches offer a rich tapestry of research opportunities, catering to diverse interests and career aspirations within the pharmaceutical field.

1.2 Understanding research: Going beneath the surface

Deliberate studies utilizing a scientific approach (quantitative, qualitative, experimental, observation, etc.) to address a pressing issue and provide new or additional knowledge are referred to as research. A third definition of research is an investigation into the reality of something, leading to the testing of theories, the addressing of queries, the formulation of new ones, the discovery of answers, and the production of new knowledge. Other researchers must be able to challenge, reuse, and apply this new knowledge. Validity (a logical process to answer a question), dependability (quality of measurement), and unbiased conclusion (exact measures are taken to ensure that it is free from individual interest) are just a few of the challenging exams that a piece of exploration must pass through to be classified as research. As a result, a PhD study needs to meet the prerequisites listed above for a scientific research protocol. (7). The study needs to clarify the uniqueness of the issue and show how critical thinking and analytical abilities are applied to support or refute the issue. It must describe how the issue will be resolved and how the knowledge gap will be closed. A well-written project provides a rationale for selecting the specific approach and discusses the appropriate methodology employed to conduct the investigation (8). A research project needs to provide answers to the following questions, as the discussion above makes clear:

- *What am I going to do?*
- *Who has conducted comparable studies?*
- *What are the findings?*

• *How will I implement this study?*

• *What makes this study particularly noteworthy?*

Lastly, your references must contain well-selected scholarly articles that deal with the same topic.

1.3 Strategies to select an effective research topic

Selecting a perfect topic for a doctoral thesis or dissertation is arguably one of graduate students' most significant choices. Before deciding on a good topic for their dissertation, some postgraduate students may search for possible subjects for a year or longer. Choosing a study topic requires making many decisions, which can be time-consuming and frustrating. Yet, regardless of the student's academic discipline, several effective methods exist for locating such a topic. While choosing a study topic entails determining the most important aspects and comparing their value against the many options accessible, finding a research topic involves looking at many sorts of literature (9). Hence, this section briefly describes various approaches to finding and choosing an ideal research topic for PhD scholars.

1.3.1   Generate ideas for potential research topics

Creative thinking is required to develop novel, inventive, and distinctive ideas. The following are a few sources for research topics:

a) *Search the internet, but be careful:* Not every website is trustworthy and secure. Try to avoid non-trustworthy websites.

b) *Build an academic network within and outside the university:* It's not necessary to choose a topic on your own. The researcher can network with senior citizens, teachers, and other students to generate creative ideas. Try to visit local academic and research institutions to learn about the work being done by others.

c) ***Attend as many viva-voce***: As much as feasible since the conversations that take place during an oral dissertation defence could reveal novel fields of interest.

d) ***Check the thrust areas for research:*** Examine the trust sections of websites belonging to international funding agencies, relevant ministries/departments, and universities of interest. A well-crafted proposal from the sponsor's areas of interest stands a higher possibility of being awarded a fully financed project or scholarship.

e) ***Find out the industries' problems:*** Ideas for finding solutions to problems can win fully Industry-funded research.

f) ***Organize brainstorming sessions:*** Organize brainstorming sessions with 4-6 knowledgeable people and consider the ideas generated.

g) ***A good research idea*** may arise from Certain circumstances or events in the outside world that can give a brilliant study concept. For instance, COVID-19 has made it possible to research the socioeconomic, clinical, immunological, pathological, microbiological, and preventative aspects of the pandemic (10,11).

1.3.2 The essence of topic selection and trends

The essence of the topic selection criteria is encapsulated in the acronym FRIENDS, which is created by employing the word's initial letter (Image 1.1). Additional words or phrases on the right that correspond to these terms provide pointers to each word's specifics.

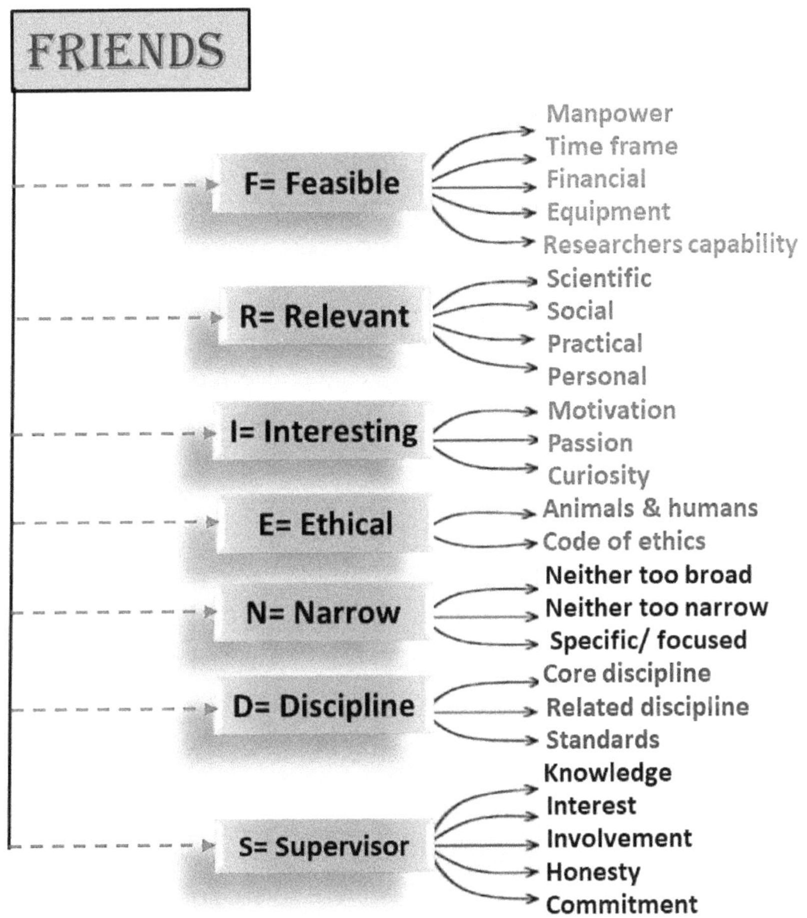

Image 1.1: Suggested framework for topic selection.

1.3.3   Converting ideas into research topics

After coming up with ideas, researchers must critically assess those ideas to identify possible research topics. The following methods are used in this process:

a) Identify your passion and interest

Choosing a research topic driven by interest and passion has several advantages, such as long-term commitment, increased research contributions, improved creativity, sustained motivation, personal fulfilment, and career alignment. Pursuing research that aligns with your interests and enthusiasm can fully realise your doctorate research potential and allow you to make significant contributions to your field of study.

b) Feasibility of the resources and facilities

The viability of proposed themes must be evaluated, as must the project's ability to be completed with the available funds, labour, time, equipment, and other resources. Studies in research have a time limit. Uncertainties can occasionally arise for researchers and have an impact on project timelines. One PhD project involved a researcher who wasted a year getting and repairing equipment since the leading equipment was not functioning correctly. Consequently, the project took four years to complete instead of three years. In turn, the investigator can evaluate their SWOT (strengths, weaknesses, opportunities, and threats). The researcher might have to step outside of their comfort zone and pick up new abilities if the issue does not align with their strengths in terms of training and experience (12).

c) Scientific, practical, social, or personal relevance

It is imperative that the subject matter be relevant to science, society, or practice, or that it benefit other scholars, practitioners, and researchers. It needs to fit a researcher's professional objectives. Ideally, the topic's research will add something novel to the discipline. Before

Submitting their PhD dissertation, most colleges require candidates to publish two or three papers in reputable publications to prove their original and novel research effort. Research can be done to address real-world issues in businesses or organizations. If the industry will benefit from the predicted study, they will be interested and willing to sponsor it. Research needs to be pertinent to the societies or communities in which it is carried out (13).

d) Conduct a literature review

A literature study establishes the current state of knowledge, the quality of the existing knowledge, and potential directions for future research. A literature review contributes to advancing knowledge in a correlated topic. You might pick up knowledge of key ideas, investigations, and testing strategies utilized in the pharmaceutical industry. Additionally, you can learn how scholars use the ideas to address issues in the actual world (14).

e) Identify and consult with peers & mentors

There are many benefits to consulting peers and mentors when choosing a research topic, such as access to a variety of viewpoints, professional advice, networking opportunities, supportive feedback, constructive criticism, idea validation, resource availability, and opportunities for both personal and professional development. Working together improves the Caliber of your study and solidifies your standing as an authority in the academic community. A matrix for selecting a topic and a mentor that takes the candidate's interest in the subject and the guidance of an advisor into account is shown in Image 1.2. The ideal choice is found in

Quadrant I (mentoring), where the scholar and the guide are both very knowledgeable about the subject. If the researcher can work alone with little assistance from the Guide, then Quadrant II (coaching) is the next best option. An apprenticeship in Quadrant III is not a wise choice. The PhD student might not attempt to work independently because they rely on their supervisor's experience. Quadrant IV is not recommended because the guide is not very involved and the scholar is not interested in the subject. There are instances where PhD students are taken advantage of by their mentors. Thus, before appointing someone as the supervisor, attempt to learn about their past performance as a faculty member (15).

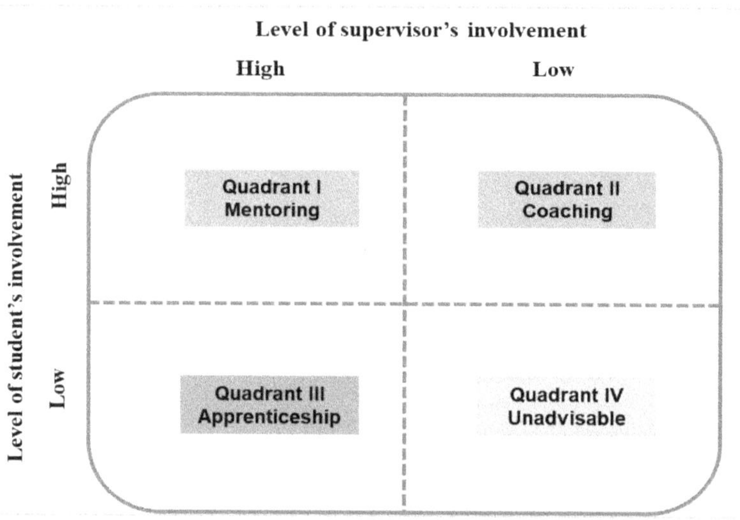

Image 1.2: Choosing a topic and an adviser matrix.

f)   Narrow down the broad topic to a specific topic

Research will be challenging to undertake when a topic's scope is too broad or too limited. Due to time and resource constraints, if the topic is too broad, the researcher is likely to write only in general and not go deeply into the issue. A topic that is too restricted will make it more difficult to locate relevant material needed to outline the study's history and pinpoint a research gap. The broad subject must be reduced to a focused area appropriate for further study (16).Let's use *"Recent trends of medical treatment in India"* as our study topic. For a focused study, it is either too general or too broad, and it might not be feasible for a researcher to cover every sector in the allotted time and financial limits. The subject matter may be narrowed down to the mining industry, and then even more narrowly to *"Recent trends of immunotherapy for cancer."* It can also be limited to specific medicinal interventions, like immunotherapy. The process of increasingly focusing on a single topic—*"Recent trends of immunotherapy for lung cancer"*—is depicted in Image 1.3. We have not diminished its significance by limiting the scope; instead, we have made it appropriate for a targeted investigation that makes sense.

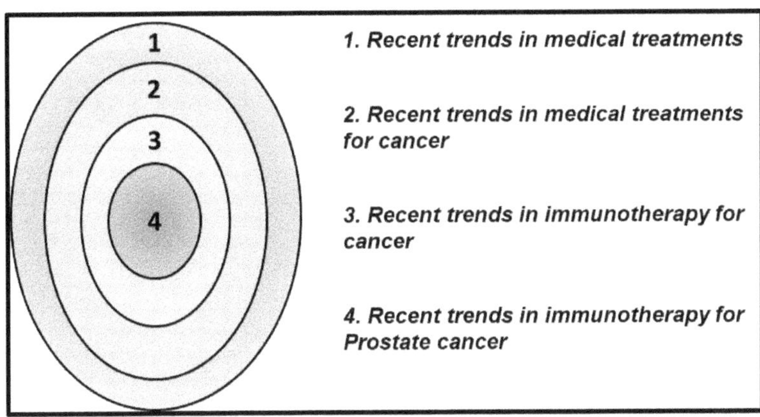

Image 1.3: Converting a broad topic to a narrow topic by restricting certain parameters.

g) Overlook of official networking platforms

LinkedIn or ResearchGate can be innovative approaches that allow you to leverage your network and access diverse perspectives.

- **Identify relevant contacts:** Find LinkedIn contacts employed in your sector of interest or possess subject-matter expertise relevant to your research. Professionals, scholars, professors, business executives, and industry specialists can all be found among these contacts.

- **Join relevant groups and communities:** Become a member of LinkedIn groups or other social media platforms associated with your area of interest or study. Engage in conversations, exchange perspectives, and establish connections with like-minded people who could provide insightful commentary on possible research subjects.

- **Engage in conversations and polls**: Use social networking sites like LinkedIn to start discussions, surveys, or polls on possible study subjects. To determine interest and spot new trends or areas of interest, pose questions, get answers, and compile feedback from your network.

- **ResearchGate:** Researchgate.net is a social networking site created for scientists and academics to exchange and collaborate on scholarly projects. (researchgate.net/).

h) Attend academic conferences and seminars

Choosing a research topic can be significantly aided by attending academic conferences, seminars, and workshops, which offer opportunities for networking with peers and specialists as well as exposure to current research trends. In addition, it offers access to specialized workshops and sessions, a look at research methodologies, a conversation about opportunities and challenges in research, a display of state-of-the-art tools and technologies, an assessment of the possible impact of the research, and motivation from influential keynote speakers (17).

i)   Search the topic by using artificial intelligence (AI) tools

For a long time, social media has been extensively utilized in education. The quick growth of AI is essential to every facet of education system learning and knowledge acquisition. Well-known AI systems like ChatGPT, Research Rabbit, and Gemini have made research direction decisions, found new research opportunities, and expedited the topic selection process. In addition, PhD holders and students can use these tools to further their research endeavours by utilizing the insightful insights they offer (18).

j)   Search engine and databases

Search engines can be invaluable tools for selecting a research topic by providing access to vast amounts of information and scholarly resources. Using search engines, you can find current concerns, rising trends, and gaps in the literature that could inspire new study subjects. Scientific information on doing literature reviews in various disciplines of study to counteract biased assumptions such as unscientific comparisons and unfounded recommendations may be found in researcher databases. These databases are presented in several steps: finding, recognizing, reading, summarizing, assembling, evaluating, interpreting, and citing (19). Table 1.1 mentions the standard search engines and databases frequently used in pharmaceutical PhD programs.

Table 1.1: Professional search engines to explore a research topic.

Search engine	Significance	Websites
Google Scholar	It provides full text or metadata of scholarly research. It is a vast repository of academic papers, theses, books, conference proceedings, and other scholarly materials.	Google Scholar
PubMed	PubMed is a free search engine that mainly retrieves references and abstracts on biomedical and life sciences subjects from the Medline database. Researchers in biology, medicine, and allied fields can benefit from it.	PubMed
JSTOR	University organizations can use JSTOR, an online library, to store and manage their intellectual works. Its extensive collection of scholarly publications, books, and sources from several fields makes it a valuable resource for multidisciplinary research.	JSTOR
Scopus	Scopus is a compilation of references and summaries from various academic disciplines. It aids in identifying writers, understanding the significance of various papers, and determining who mentions researchers' work.	Scopus
BASE	BASE is a large search engine that finds a wide range of Academic material online. It searches open-access websites and	BASE

	journals for papers and articles on many different subjects.	
Microsoft Academic	Academic papers, conference proceedings, and patents can all be found in the index of Microsoft Academic, a freely available academic search engine. It helps academics find pertinent literature and spot research trends with its sophisticated search capabilities and citation analysis features.	Microsoft Academic
EBSCOhost	It is a collection of databases covering a wide range of topics, such as business, education, healthcare, and academic research. It provides access to full-text articles, abstracts, and other academic materials.	EBSCOhost

Other online platforms: With its instructional channels, tutorials, and scholarly lectures, YouTube is an excellent tool for PhD thesis writers. Researchers can use these materials to investigate different fields, understand possible research subjects more deeply, and comprehend complex ideas. Furthermore, YouTube offers a forum for exchanging research techniques and insights, cultivating a community of academics who participate in discussions and presentations to influence the selection of topics (youtube.com).

1.4 References

1. Bernery C, Lusardi L, Marino C, Philippe-Lesaffre M, Angulo E, Bonnaud E, et al. Highlighting the positive aspects of being a PhD student. eLife. 2022 Jul 26;11: e81075.
2. Mosanya AU, Ukoha-kalu BO, Isah A, Umeh I, Amorha KC, Ayogu EE, et al. Factors associated with the timely completion of doctoral research studies in clinical pharmacy: A mixed-methods study. Chaudhary P, editor. PLoS ONE. 2022 Sep 30;17(9): e0274638.
3. Alsultan A, Alghamdi WA, Alghamdi J, Alharbi AF, Aljutayli A, Albassam A, et al. Clinical pharmacology applications in clinical drug development and clinical care: A focus on Saudi Arabia. Saudi Pharmaceutical Journal. 2020 Oct;28(10):1217–27.
4. Grogan S, Preuss CV. Pharmacokinetics. Treasure Island (FL): StatPearls Publishing [Internet]. 2023; Available from: https://www.ncbi.nlm.nih.gov/books/NBK557744/
5. Hassan M, Sallam H, Hassan Z. The Role of Pharmacokinetics and Pharmacodynamics in Early Drug Development concerning the Cyclin-dependent Kinase (CDK) Inhibitor - Roscovitine. Sultan Qaboos Univ Med J. 2011 May;11(2):165–78.
6. Orhan IE. Pharmacognosy: Science of natural products in drug discovery. Bioimpacts. 2017 Aug 23;4(3):109–10.
7. Faryadi, Q. How to write your PhD proposal: A step-by-step guide. AIJCR. 2012;2(4):111–5.
8. Boudah D. Conducting Educational Research: Guide to Completing a Major Project [Internet]. 2455 Teller Road, Thousand Oaks California 91320 United States: SAGE Publications, Inc.; 2011 [cited 2024 Mar 19]. Available from: https://sk.sagepub.com/books/conducting-educational-research
9. Lei, Simon A. Strategies for finding and selecting an ideal thesis or dissertation topic: a literature review. College Student Journal. 2009;43(4):1324.
10. Wang GT, Park K. Student research and report writing: from topic selection to the complete paper. West Sussex; Malden, MA: Wiley Blackwell; 2016. 267 p.
11. Roberts CM. The dissertation journey: a practical and comprehensive guide to planning, writing, and defending your dissertation. 2nd ed. Thousand Oaks, Calif: Corwin Press; 2010. 229 p.
12. Du JT, Evans N. Academic Users' Information Searching on Research Topics: Characteristics of Research Tasks and Search Strategies. The Journal of Academic Librarianship. 2011 Jul;37(4):299–306.

13. Okpala HN, Benneh EA, Sefu A, Kalule E. Advancing the Information Literacy Skills of Postgraduate Students in University of Nigeria. 2017;

14. Reviewing the literature: a critical review. University of Melbourne. 2013;

15. Martin B. Countering Supervisor Exploitation. Journal of Scholarly Publishing. 2013 Oct;45(1):74–86.

16. Adhikari DGR. Strategies for Selecting a Research Topic. 2020;22(1).

17. Hauss K. What are the social and scientific benefits of participating in academic conferences? Insights from a survey among doctoral students and postdocs in Germany. Research Evaluation. 2021 Oct 7;30(1):1–12.

18. Piercy H, Gordon F. Different but the Same: Doctoral Students' Experience of Multiprofessional Education. Education. 2015 Mar 13;3(4):393–8.

19. Chigbu UE, Atiku SO, Du Plessis CC. The Science of Literature Reviews: Searching, Identifying, Selecting, and Synthesising. Publications. 2023 Jan 6;11(1):2.

Chapter 2

SYNOPSIS PREPARATION

Creating new knowledge is the essence of research.

2.1 Overview

A synopsis should be a short, systematic outline of your proposed thesis, made in preparation for your first meeting with your supervisor. It ensures that your supervisor gets a clear picture of the proposed project and allows them to spot gaps or things you have yet to consider. The synopsis is structured into several sections, each addressing a specific aspect and outlining the research's focus areas and key components to obtain approval. The synopsis contains different headlines, just like the chapters in PhD thesis writing, to clearly discuss all those areas and is submitted separately at the beginning of your research.

Sometimes, a thesis synopsis is referred to as a research proposal. However, there can be slight differences in their purposes and formats depending on academic institutions or disciplines (1). A thesis synopsis usually includes a summary of the main points of the thesis, including the significance, predicted results, methodology, and research aims. A thesis summary, to put it simply, is a shortened version of the thesis that is frequently used for assessment or presentation (2). A research proposal, on the other hand, is a detailed document that describes how a research project will be carried out. Background data, research questions or hypotheses, a literature review, methodology, a schedule, and a budget are typically included (3) Research proposals are frequently used to request approval from academic supervisors or review committees, apply for financing, or both (4).

2.2 Purpose of Synopsis Writing

- **Clarity and focus:** The research scope is made clear, which is the main emphasis of the summary.

- **Assessment and approval:** It facilitates the assessment and approval of the suggested work by supervisors.

- **Communication:** A synopsis effectively conveys the goals of the investigation.

- **Planning and organization:** It facilitates the planning and setup of the study endeavour.

- **Reference and documentation:** The research is referenced and documented in the synopsis.

- **Revision and feedback:** It starts the process of revision and feedback for enhancement.

2.3 Understanding the University Guidelines

The term "university guidelines" refers to the set of regulations, directives, expectations, and standards that an academic institution issues to control several facets of academic activity, such as teaching, research, and administrative processes. These principles guarantee quality, uniformity, and adherence to academic standards in all of the university's programs and disciplines. PhD candidates and postgraduate researchers should check if their synopsis satisfies university standards by speaking with their advisors or supervisors. Supervisors can offer insightful direction and explanation on policies specific to the university (5).

University rules should specify students' expectations regarding formatting a thesis or synopsis, citation styles, academic integrity, ethical research practices, admissions processes, grading criteria, and graduation requirements. The university's instructors, staff, administrators, and students can refer to these principles, which are usually recorded in official publications like handbooks, manuals, regulations, or web pages. University guidelines would outline the precise structure, content, and submission procedures that PhD applicants should adhere to while developing and submitting their synopsis for review and approval in the context of a PhD. This policy is readily available for download on the college's or university's official website.As an illustration, visit https://www.bnuniversity.ac.in/Research for postgraduate studies at Bhupal Nobles' University, Udaipur, 313001 (Raj).

2.4 Effective synopsis construction

The synopsis for PhD students can be divided into the following sections. Your synopsis might have additional sections, depending on discipline and the type of research you are conducting.

2.4.1 Page setup and layout

Writing a synopsis requires careful consideration of page organization and style to ensure the text is well-structured, aesthetically pleasing, and easy to navigate. Paper size, margins, font style, size, colour, line spacing, page number, header & footer, paragraph alignment, headers, and subheadings are a few of the essential factors it takes into account (6).

2.4.2 Cover page/ title page

The title page includes essential details, including the research project's title, the researcher's name, affiliation, registration number, supervisor's name, and the submission date. The format of the title page follows the criteria set by the institution. The primary goal of the research should be brief and conveyed in the title, which should also be unique (7).

Research title: Development and Characterization of Second Generation PAMAM Dendrimers to Increase the Bioavailability of Efavirenz.

Image 2.1: Example of title.

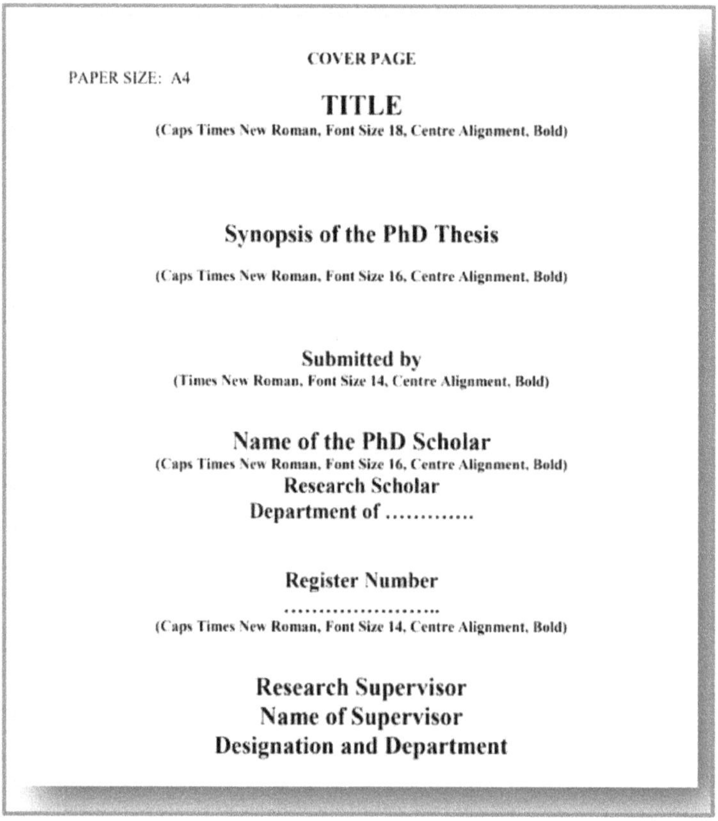

COVER PAGE

PAPER SIZE: A4

TITLE
(Caps Times New Roman, Font Size 18, Centre Alignment, Bold)

Synopsis of the PhD Thesis

(Caps Times New Roman, Font Size 16, Centre Alignment, Bold)

Submitted by
(Times New Roman, Font Size 14, Centre Alignment, Bold)

Name of the PhD Scholar
(Caps Times New Roman, Font Size 16, Centre Alignment, Bold)
Research Scholar
Department of ....

Register Number
....
(Caps Times New Roman, Font Size 14, Centre Alignment, Bold)

Research Supervisor
Name of Supervisor
Designation and Department

Image 2.2: Cover page.

2.4.3   Index

Provide a table listing the main summary sections, subsections, and corresponding page numbers. This will facilitate readers' effective navigation of your document.

CHAPTER	CONTENT	PAGE NO.
1	INTRODUCTION	2 – 10
2	REVIEW OF LITERATURE	11 – 17
3	AIM, OBJECTIVES & NEED OF THE STUDY	18 – 19
4	PLAN OF WORK	19 – 20
5	MATERIALS AND METHODS	20 – 24
6	EXPECTED OUTCOMES	24
7	REFERENCE	24 – 30
	LIST OF PUBLICATIONS	30

Image 2.3: Content/ index page.

2.4.4   Introduction

A research introduction is the first part of a research summary or any document that presents the subject, gives background knowledge, and establishes the context for the investigation. This is your chance to demonstrate to the reader of your research topic in the first section of the main text (8). It ought to be clear and evocative. It needs to be engaging and educational. Depending on the requirements set forth by the university, the introduction may be up to 2000 words. A strong opening gets the reader interested and leans them in the direction of the proposal (9). Thus, the crucial steps of writing the introduction are described below.

- *Step 1: Introduce your topic*

State the main focus and highlight. Also, mention why it is exciting or essential.

- *Step 2: Describe the background*

Briefly summarise the main ideas, theories, or earlier studies pertinent to the study question.

- *Step 3: Establish your research problem*

Clarify the precise research questions or objectives that the study seeks to answer and point out any gaps or weaknesses in the body of current knowledge.

- *Step 4: Specify your objective(s)*

Indicate the study's purpose or research objectives in clear terms.

- *Step 5: Identify the research gap*

Determine the void or shortcoming in the present body of literature that the research fills. Describe the need for the research and how it will close the knowledge or understanding gap. The visibility and impact of the synopsis can be increased by including visual components in the study introduction, such as photographs, tables, and scientific procedures.

Following these guidelines, you can write a study summary's beginning section successfully.

2.4.5   Aim & Objectives

The goal of a summary is to provide the reader with a thorough, concise overview of the entire work so they can understand its main ideas without having to read it themselves. Conversely, objectives set precise goals to be met to fulfil the aims. Give a clear explanation of your study's overall goal and particular targets. What do you want your research to accomplish? Your goals should be SMART (Image 2.4) (2).

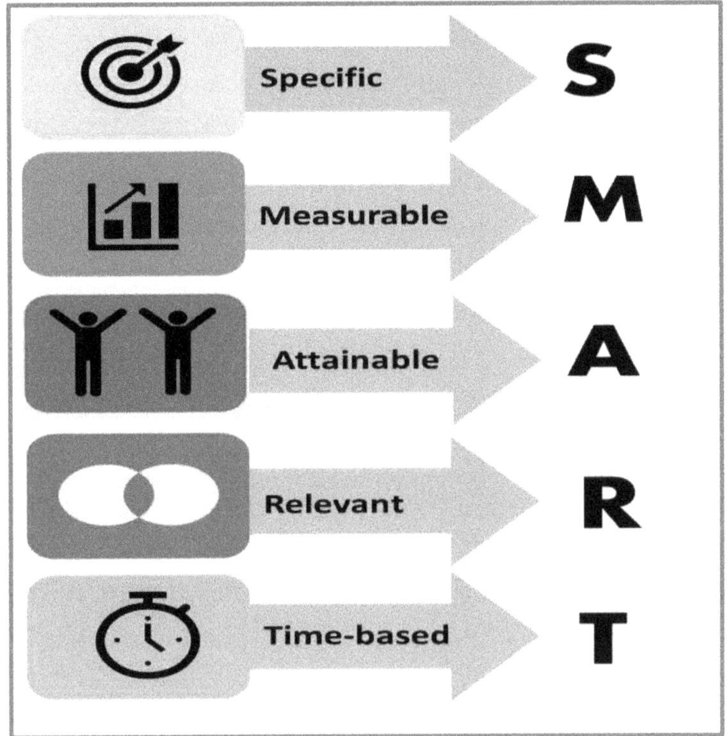

Image 2.4: Specifications for objectives.

2.4.6   Need / rationale of the study

Research rationales are justifications for undertaking research generally or focusing on a specific problem, objective, or question. (10). Justify your approach choices' suitability for achieving your research goals or questions. Consider any possible restrictions and your strategy for minimizing them.

2.4.7   Literature review

A summary of the previously published works on a topic is what a literature review is. Make a thorough analysis of the body of knowledge already available on the subject of your study. Discuss essential ideas, theories, research techniques, conclusions, and arguments. Point out any gaps or areas that require more study. The student should do relevant research before writing this section by looking for relevant publications online and in libraries, scientific journals, databases, and other online resources. Additionally, seek assistance from mentors, more experienced students, and others engaged in the field or subject of study that has been chosen. However, while choosing, analyzing, and incorporating pertinent research papers, the student needs to exercise critical thinking. It is advised that before beginning to write a summary and have copies, student(s) read at least 15-20 original research publications (11).

2.4.8   Plan of Work

The plan of work or research plan serves as a roadmap for researchers to follow throughout their study, ensuring that they stay focused and organized while pursuing their research goals (9). In the research synopsis, provide an overview of your targeted methodology and plan and a description of the study design, data collection strategies, analytic methodologies, and other pertinent information.

Give a timetable or timeline outlining the steps you plan to take to complete each study phase.

2.4.9   Methodology

The method section is vital because it tells your research committee how you plan to tackle your research problem. It outlines the equipment and procedures that helped you accomplish the goals mentioned in the Introduction. Depending on the area and journal, the Methods section may also be referred to as Materials and Methods, Procedures, Methodology, Experiments, or other comparable terms. The drafting of the methods section should be guided by the goal of providing the reader with enough information to assess the soundness of the methodology (12). This part should provide detailed experimental protocols, analytical processes, and statistical methodologies that must be used. Relevant and reliable literature citations should back each up. The talk with a statistician during the experiment planning phase is one area that is frequently disregarded, even though it is essential and beneficial for both students and supervisors. The research facilities offered by the university, sister institutes, or student departments where the requirements might be fulfilled are another essential factor to consider (13).

2.4.10 *Expected outcomes*

Expected outcomes are also called forecasted results. Discuss the anticipated outcomes of your research. For example,

- What do you hope to discover or achieve?
- How will your research add to the corpus of information already known about pharmaceutical sciences?

Be realistic but also highlight the potential significance of your work (14).(Image 2.5).

For example, if we have chosen to prepare and assess nanoparticles, the anticipated results should meet the ideal standards for size, pre-formulation, and other factors.

Expected outcomes

i.   Pre-formulation analysis of drug and excipients must comply with the reference value regarding melting point, UV, FTIR, etc.

ii. Drugs must be compatible with excipients, and it will be confirmed by a rug-excipients compatibility study.

iii. Size of Nanoparticles determines the distribution, stability, and uptake of drug. Hence, zeta potential, PDI, vesicle size must be in optimum range.

iv. Drug content, entrapment efficiency, and loading capacity should significantly increase.

v.   Stability study should not report any changes in the final formulation.

Image 2.5: Example of expected outcomes.

2.4.11   References

Provide a list of all the references your summary cites. Finding the sources used should be easy for the reader thanks to a reference list. Different referencing styles exist (APA, MLA, Chicago, Vancouver, etc.). Observe the citation format that your discipline or university specifies. Make sure that every reference is valid and appropriately formatted (15).

Example of Vancouver referencing style

Alsultan A, Alghamdi WA, Alghamdi J, Alharbi AF, Aljutayli A, Albassam A, et al. Clinical pharmacology applications in clinical drug development and clinical care: A focus on Saudi Arabia. Saudi Pharmaceutical Journal. 2020 Oct;28(10):1217–27.

Image 2.6: Example of reference.

2.4.12   List of publications

Provide a list of all the publications (journal articles, conference papers, etc.) that came about as a result of your study or related projects, if applicable. Give each publication's complete bibliographic information.

2.5 Revising, final editing, proofreading, and submission

This crucial stage ensures that the summary accurately captures the main ideas of the study, follows the rules, and conveys the importance of the work. Revision entails improving language, making ideas more understandable, and responding to criticism. The final editing phase carefully examines Every synopsis element for accuracy, coherence, and consistency. After that, proofreading is done with an emphasis on removing syntax, grammar, and punctuation mistakes to improve readability and professionalism. The result of all of this work is the production of a polished study summary that is prepared for review and dissemination (16).

2.6 Synopsis presentation

Once the synopsis for the pharmacy Ph.D. thesis has been completed, making an impactful, informative, and clear presentation is essential once the synopsis for the pharmacy PhD thesis has been completed. When creating a summary presentation, follow the institutional guidelines. For instance, PhD presentations at Dow University of Health Sciences (DUHS) are limited to a maximum of 15 slides.

2.6.1   *Essential contents in presentation*

First, make sure you fully comprehend the synopsis's contents. Next, begin with a clear, evocative title that appropriately summarizes your findings. Briefly summarize the research problem, its importance, and your goals in the introduction. The literature review provides an overview of pertinent material while pointing out knowledge gaps. Explain your research approach and why it is appropriate for your research issue. Give an accurate timeframe for finishing each study phase and an explanation of the anticipated results and their importance. Determine the resources that are required and take any ethical issues into account. Calculate how much money will be needed for the research. Summarize the main ideas and highlight the significance of your research in your conclusion. Before beginning your actual study, get input from your supervisor or peers on the synopsis and make any necessary modifications (17,18).

2.7 References

1.   Larsen HO. Research synopsis writing.
2.   Betkerur J. Guidelines for writing a research project synopsis or protocol. Indian J Dermatol Venereol Leprol. 2008;74(6):687.
3.   Abdulai RT, Owusu-Ansah A. Essential Ingredients of a Good Research Proposal for Undergraduate and Postgraduate Students in the Social Sciences. SAGE Open. 2014 Jul 1;4(3):215824401454817.

4. Setia MS, Panda S. Summary and Synthesis: How to Present a Research Proposal. Indian J Dermatol. 2017;62(5):443–50.

5. Ghafoor, Abdul. Manual for Synopsis and Thesis Preparation. Univ of Agri, Faislabad, Pakistan 68P. 2007;

6. Schwen LO. Ten simple rules for typographically appealing scientific texts. Markel S, editor. PLoS Comput Biol. 2020 Dec 31;16(12):e1008458.

7. Du JT, Evans N. Academic Users' Information Searching on Research Topics: Characteristics of Research Tasks and Search Strategies. The Journal of Academic Librarianship. 2011 Jul;37(4):299–306.

8. Larsen HO. Research synopsis guidelines. 2015 [cited 2024 Mar 20]; Available from: http://rgdoi.net/10.13140/RG.2.1.3478.3840

9. Wong P. How to write a research proposal. International network on Personal meaning. 2008; Available from: www.meaning.ca/archives

10. Younas A, Durante A, Fàbregues S. Understanding the Nature of and Identifying and Formulating "Research Problems" in Mixed Methods Research. Journal of Mixed Methods Research. 2023 Jul 25;15586898231191441.

11. Roberts CM. The dissertation journey: a practical and comprehensive guide to planning, writing, and defending your dissertation. 2nd ed. Thousand Oaks, Calif: Corwin Press; 2010. 229 p.

12. Al-Riyami A. How to prepare a Research Proposal. Oman Med J. 2008 Apr;23(2):66–9.

13. Erdemir F. How to write a materials and methods section of a scientific article? Turkish Journal of Urology. 2014 Oct 15;39(1):10–5.

14. Pat Cryer. The Research Student's Guide to Success. In Taiwan: International Forum of Educational Technology & Society, National Taiwan Normal University; 2007.

15. Januszewicz, Wladyslaw. Study Synopsis.

16. Revising, Editing, and Proofreading University of Toronto Faculty of Applied Science and Engineering.

17. Paun, Ms Jalpa S., And Drhm Tank. PH. D. Synopsis. 2016;

18. Bashir A. Synopsis of PhD Thesis. IETE Technical Review. 1984 Aug;1(8):130–130.

Chapter 3

LITERATURE SURVEY

Exploring the past to illuminate the present.

3.1 Purpose of conducting a literature review

An essential component of academic research is the literature review. It serves as a lighthouse, directing scholars over the vast sea of existing knowledge (1). It entails carefully examining what prior research has found for a particular subject. But why is it so important? Why should we put in the time and energy to do that? Consider it this way: before constructing a new home, you should be aware of the materials that are now in stock and the designs that have already been attempted. The same goes for research. Researchers can obtain a clear picture of what has already been investigated, what questions have been addressed, and what gaps need to be filled by performing a literature survey. It's similar to setting the framework for your research (2). But it is not just about gathering information.

The literature reviews are essential for the following:

- Identifying what has been written on a subject or topic (3).
- Identifying topics or questions requiring further research.
- Developing new frameworks and theories.
- Assessing the degree to which a particular research area reveals any interpretable trends or patterns.
- Compiling empirical findings relevant to a specific research question to support evidence-based practice (4).

A well-structured literature review should have three main components at minimum: an introduction or background information section that provides context and highlights the review's focus; the review's body that discusses sources chronologically, methodologically, or thematically; and, lastly, a conclusion and/or recommendations section that highlights the main conclusions and makes recommendations for additional research (5).

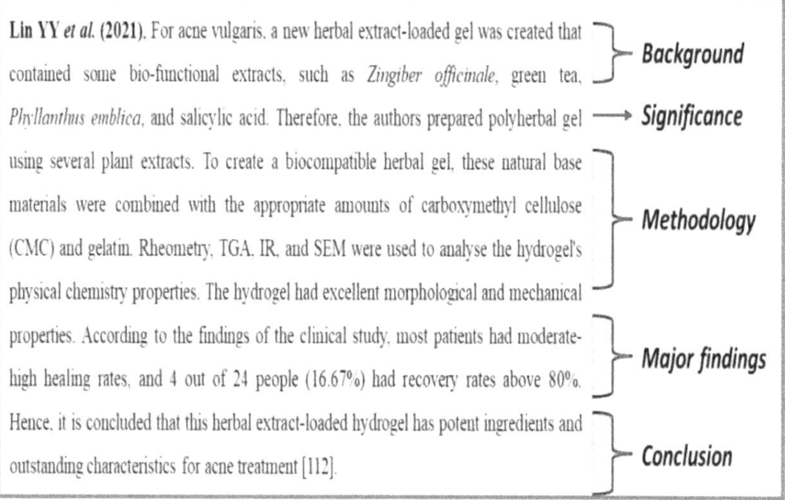

Image 3.1: Components of literature review.

Researchers and PhD holders, through their innovative strategies, are significantly advancing their fields by synthesizing all available knowledge. The literature review, a crucial stage, lays the foundation for impactful scientific investigation. It's not just a compass in the desert of research; it's a powerful tool you can use to substantially contribute to your field. Embrace, investigate, and let it guide you in writing a compelling doctoral thesis. (6). Here, we have discussed 10 rules as a quick guide for doing literature.

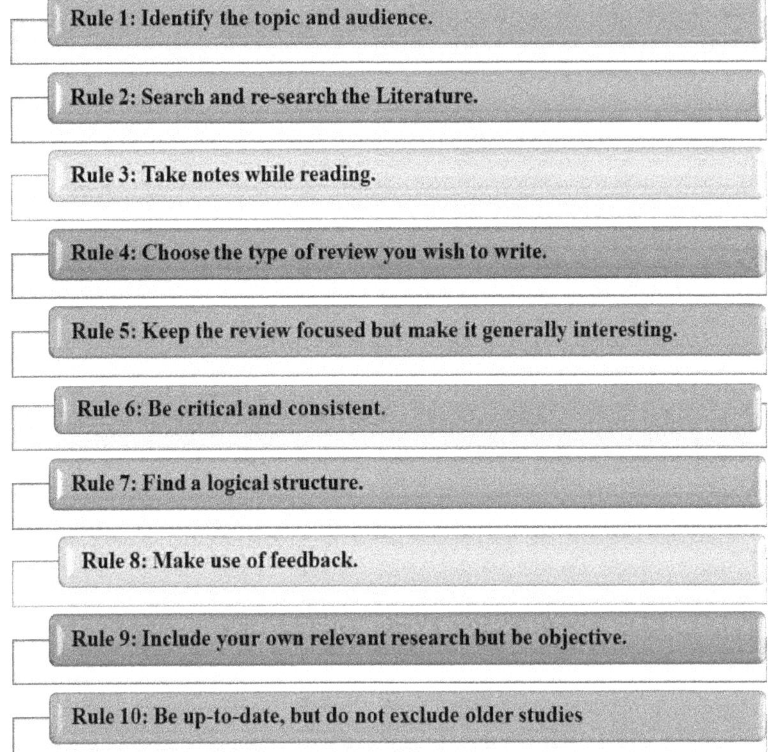

Image 3.2: Ten rules of literature review (Own creation).

3.2 Sources of literature review

- **Primary sources:** Original research studies, reports, or publications that give firsthand information, data, or experimental results from scholarly or scientific research are referred to as primary literature sources.

Examples: Research articles, clinical trials, case studies, dissertations, theses, conference proceedings, patents, and technical reports.

- **Secondary sources:** Works that evaluate, interpret, comment on, or condense original materials or previous study findings are called secondary literature.

Examples: Review articles, textbooks, encyclopedias, meta-analyses, commentaries, and critical essays.

- **Tertiary Source:** The sources that make up tertiary literature combine and compress data from primary and secondary sources, frequently displaying it in an easier-to-read manner.

Examples: The Encyclopaedias of Psychology, textbook glossaries, manuals, handbooks, etc (7).

3.3 Approaches for conducting a literature review

3.3.1   *Read research manuscripts, books, review articles, and magazines related to the topic*

An essential part of research for a PhD thesis is reading a wide range of literature. This includes reading articles from journals, books, reviews, and research documents pertinent to the subject of choice. Research publications provide thorough explanations of particular investigations and their conclusions, offering insightful perspectives on the most recent advancements in research. Books provide thorough coverage of a subject, including in-depth debates, hypotheses, and analyses that might broaden one's comprehension. For example, the E-book database: **Access Pharmacy-** Provides access to textbooks such as *Applied Clinical Pharmacokinetics, Basic & Clinical Pharmacology, Medication Therapy Management: A Comprehensive Approach, Toxicology: The Basic Science of Poisons, The*

Pharmacological Basis of Therapeutics, Poisoning & Drug Overdose, Pharmacotherapy: A Pathophysiologic Approach, Toxicologic Emergencies. Review articles summarize and synthesize existing literature on a particular subject, making them invaluable for gaining a broad perspective and identifying key themes. While less scholarly, magazines often contain articles and editorials that highlight current trends, debates, and issues in the field. Through exploring these diverse literature sources, researchers can gather a rich array of information, perspectives, and ideas that inform and shape their research endeavours (8).

3.3.2   *Retrieve data using search engines*

Finding relevant material online is an essential first step in any research literature survey. A wide range of scholarly literature can be accessed through well-known search engines such as Google Scholar, PubMed, Embase, Cochrane Library, Scopus, Web of Science (WoS), ScienceDirect, and others. With the help of these platforms, researchers can enter keywords associated with their area of interest and obtain pertinent papers, studies, articles, and fast communications from various sources. **Google Scholar** is a freely accessible web search engine that indexes the full text or metadata of scholarly literature across various publishing formats and disciplines. **PubMed®** is a free database comprising more than 36 million citations for biomedical literature from MEDLINE, life science journals, and online books. **Embase** is a biomedical and pharmacological bibliographic database of published literature designed in 1947. The **Cochrane Library** is a collection of databases in medicine and other healthcare specialities provided by Cochrane and other organizations. At its core is the collection of

Cochrane reviews, a database of systematic reviews and meta-analyses that summarise and interpret medical research results.

Scopus is a comprehensive, multidisciplinary, trusted abstract and citation database. The **Web of Science** is a paid-access platform that provides access to multiple databases that provide reference and citation data from academic journals, conference proceedings, and other documents in various academic disciplines. ScienceDirect covers various scientific journals and papers in disciplines, including health, engineering, and social sciences. It holds more than 18 million pieces of information from this publisher's 30,000 e-books and more than 4,000 scholarly publications. By utilising the capabilities of these search engines, scholars can effectively collect information, peruse pertinent literature, and remain informed about recent advancements in the field, thereby establishing a solid basis for their doctoral research (9,10).

3.3.3   *Utilize sci-hub to access research*

Researchers can access restricted material with the help of Sci-hub, which provides access to a wide range of scholarly journals. Given that sci-hub operates in a legal limbo by evading copyright laws, it is crucial to recognize the ethical concerns. Nevertheless, many researchers turn to sci-hub when faced with restricted access to pricey journal subscriptions. Sci-hub is a valuable tool, but to ensure a thorough and moral literature review for their PhD research thesis, scholars should also think about other ethical ways to access the literature (11).

3.3.4   *Key portals for finding research and clinical trials*

It includes vital portals like Google patents, CTRI, Clinical trials.gov, cancer.gov clinical trials, etc. The Clinical Trials Registry - India (CTRI) is a freely accessible, online public record of clinical trials conducted in India. It was established to promote transparency and accountability in clinical research and to address issues such as selective reporting and publication bias. The CTRI is maintained by the National Institute of Medical Statistics (NIMS), which is part of the Indian Council of Medical Research (ICMR). ClinicalTrials.gov is a database that houses clinical trial registrations and offers access to details about finished and ongoing trials, along with their methods and results. You may quickly retrieve the data associated with clinical studies using filters such as condition/disease, intervention/treatment, location, status, etc. The National Institutes of Health (NIH) Clinical Center, the NIH's research hospital, hosts the CCR Clinical Trials (Clinical Center Research Studies) platform. It details numerous clinical trials conducted in various medical specializations and disease areas, including observational studies, natural history investigations, and interventional trials. Google Patents provides academics with access to an extensive database of patents, allowing them to investigate cutting-edge technologies and inventions that apply to their area of study (12).

3.3.5 *Pivotal role of regulatory bodies and organization in literature surveys*

Researching regulatory organizations like the CDSCO (Central Drugs Standard Control Organization), World Health Organization (WHO), FDA (Food and Drug Administration), CDC (Centers for Disease Control and Prevention), AMA (American Medical Association), and others can be beneficial when conducting a literature review for a PhD research thesis. These regulatory agencies are essential in establishing standards, rules, and policies in the healthcare and pharmaceutical industries. Researchers can better understand safety standards, best practices, and regulatory regulations about their research themes by perusing their papers, recommendations, and reports. Indeed, these organizations provide:

- *Crucial data:* E.g., The CDC monitors the emergence and spread of COVID-19 variants, the most recent and detailed data for hospitalizations, deaths, emergency department visits, and vaccinations (https://covid.cdc.gov/covid-data-tracker/#datatracker-home).

- *Statistics:* E.g., Breast cancer caused 670,000 deaths globally in 2022 (https://www.who.int/news-room/fact-sheets/detail/breast-cancer).

- *Latest news:* E.g., **Duvyzat** is the first nonsteroidal drug approved to treat patients with all genetic variants of Duchenne muscular dystrophy (DMD), news released on March 21, 2024 (https://www.fda.gov/news-events/press-announcements/fda-approves-nonsteroidal-treatment-duchenne-muscular-dystrophy).

- *Latest update:* E.g., How AI can change health care, March 20, 2024 (https://www.ama-assn.org/). To fulfil their overarching mission of saving lives and protecting people.

The integration of perspectives from these reputable sources augments the accuracy, validity, and relevance of the study outcomes, assuring conformity with established regulatory structures and industry standards (13).

3.4 Data extraction and analysis

Data extraction is the process of carefully gathering relevant information from this research, including significant findings, methods, and conclusions; sources have been identified when possible. This data analysis combines and analyses the retrieved information to get valuable insights and pinpoint knowledge gaps. Effective literature evaluation techniques are essential for guiding pharmaceutical PhD research and guaranteeing its applicability and value to the field (14).

3.5 Constructing of literature review in a systematic format

Creating a literature review (Image 3.3) entails methodically reviewing, analyzing, and condensing previous studies and academic publications that are pertinent to your area of interest (15).

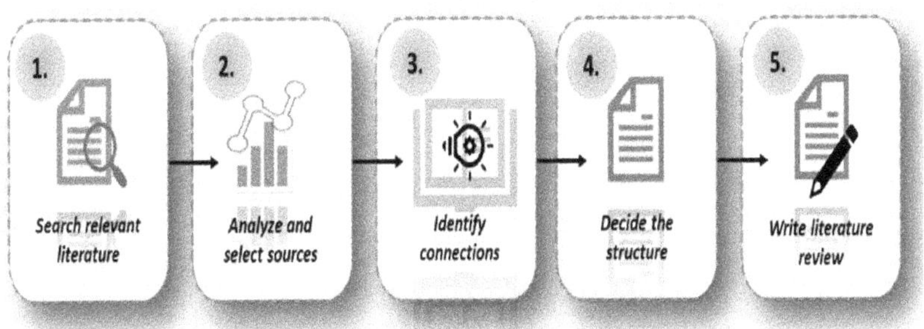

Image 3.3: Steps of constructing a literature review.

3.5.1   Writing a literature review

A PhD thesis literature evaluation requires the completion of numerous crucial tasks (16)

a) ***Introduction:*** Start your literature review by summarizing the subject and how it relates to your study. Describe the goals and parameters of your review.

b) ***Search strategy:*** Describe the methods you used to search for relevant literature. This could include databases searched, keywords used, and inclusion/exclusion criteria.

c) ***Organization:*** Organize your literature review logically. You can choose to organize it chronologically, thematically, or by methodology, depending on what best suits your research question.

d) ***Summary of studies:*** Provide a summary of each study's main conclusions that you have included in the review. Draw attention to any patterns, distinctions, or parallels between the studies.

e) ***Critical analysis:*** Critically evaluate the strengths and weaknesses of each study. Discuss any biases, limitations, or gaps in the existing literature.

f) ***Synthesis:*** Summarize the research results to derive generalizations. Talk about how the literature helps you comprehend the research question and suggest areas that need more study (Image 3.1) (17).

3.6 References

1. Fink, Arlene. Conducting Research Literature Reviews: From the Internet to Paper. United States: SAGE Publications. 2019.
2. Bruce CS. Research students' early experiences of the dissertation literature review. Studies in Higher Education. 1994 Jan;19(2):217–29.
3. Rachel Show. Conducting Literature Reviews. :39–55.
4. Paré G, Kitsiou S. Methods for Literature Reviews. In: Handbook of eHealth Evaluation: An Evidence-based Approach [Internet]. University of Victoria; 2017. Available from: https://www.ncbi.nlm.nih.gov/books/NBK481583/.
5. Literature Reviews. The University Of North Carolina At Chapel Hill.
6. Thompson P. Literature Reviews in Applied PhD Theses: Evidence and Problems. In: Hyland K, Diani G, editors. Academic Evaluation [Internet]. London: Palgrave Macmillan UK; 2009 [cited 2024 Mar 21]. p. 50–67. Available from: http://link.springer.com/10.1057/9780230244290_4.
7. Philippa Ojimelukwe. Literature Review, Overview, Sources, and Search Methods.
8. Faryadi Q. PhD Thesis Writing Process: A Systematic Approach—How to Write Your Literature Review. CE. 2018;09(16):2912–9.
9. Jesson JK. Doing your literature review: traditional and systematic techniques. London: SAGE Publications; 2012.
10. Rowley J, Slack F. Conducting a literature review. Management Research News. 2004 Jun;27(6):31–9.
11. Himmelstein DS, Romero AR, Levernier JG, Munro TA, McLaughlin SR, Greshake Tzovaras B, et al. Sci-Hub provides access to nearly all scholarly literature. eLife. 2018 Mar 1;7:e32822.
12. Bandara W, Furtmueller E, Gorbacheva E, Miskon S, Beekhuyzen J. Achieving Rigor in Literature Reviews: Insights from Qualitative Data Analysis and Tool-Support. CAIS [Internet]. 2015 [cited 2024 Mar 22];37. Available from: https://aisel.aisnet.org/cais/vol37/iss1/8/.
13. Towards a global guidance framework for the responsible use of life sciences: summary report of consultations on the principles, gaps, and challenges of risk management- World Health Organization. 2022;

14. Wang Y, Wang L, Rastegar-Mojarad M, Moon S, Shen F, Afzal N, et al. Clinical information extraction applications: A literature review. Journal of Biomedical Informatics. 2018 Jan;77:34–49.

15. Badenhorst C. Citation practices of postgraduate students writing literature reviews. London Review of Education [Internet]. 2018 [cited 2024 Mar 22];16(1). Available from: https://journals.uclpress.co.uk/lre/article/id/2861/.

16. Denney AS, Tewksbury R. How to Write a Literature Review. Journal of Criminal Justice Education. 2013 Jun;24(2):218–34.

17. Faryadi Q. PhD Thesis Writing Process: A Systematic Approach—Your Guide to Crafting Methodology, Results and Conclusion. CE. 2019; 10 (04): 766-83.

Chapter 4

RESEARCH METHODOLOGY & PLAN OF WORK

Exploring, discovering, designing: The journey of a research study.

4.1 Overview

A vital aspect of the pharmaceutical industry is research methodology (RM), which is the scientific and systematic search for relevant data on a particular subject (1). It includes the general structure, tactics, and processes researchers use to examine pharma-related subjects, produce fresh insights, and advance the discipline. It includes research types, standards, goals, and importance (2).

4.2 Selecting appropriate research methodologies

Research methodology should be rigorous, relevant, and meaningful to this domain (3).The choice of an RM is influenced by several criteria, including the nature of the research question or hypothesis, the investigator's experience, the accessibility of data and resources, ethical issues, and financing prospects (4). For instance, a randomized controlled trial may be ideal if you examine a novel medication's effectiveness. Qualitative methods can be a better fit if you want to investigate how a specific medicine has affected patients. On the other hand, when measuring relationships or phenomena with numerical data, quantitative approaches like surveys or experiments could be more appropriate. To guarantee coherence and rigour in the results, the chosen approaches should also align with the project's theoretical framework and overall study plan. As a result, thoughtful consideration and justification of RMs are crucial to the project's effective execution and significant results.

4.3 Types of research methods

a) **Descriptive research:** Surveys, observations, case studies, and other fact-finding inquiries are used in this kind of study. Its main goal is to present the current state of affairs. Another name for it is ex post facto research (5,6). It offers a thorough explanation of the topic, which makes it an invaluable tool in pharmaceutical research since comprehending the current situation is frequently the first step. One type of descriptive study describes the patterns of antibiotic prescriptions given by medical professionals in a community over a given time frame.

b) **Analytical research:** This type of research is frequently done to find data that validates and adds credibility to the research they are already doing. It's also done to generate new thoughts about the subject matter of the inquiry. In various professions, it facilitates comprehension, problem-solving, and well-informed decision-making. The facts and factual material at their disposal, which they may interpret to do a thorough analysis of the data (7,8). E.g., analyzing clinical trial data to determine the effectiveness of a new drug in treating a specific condition.

c) **Applied research:** It is a systematic and structured investigation to resolve particular issues in the real world or enhance current procedures, products, or services. In contrast to fundamental research, which aims to increase broad knowledge, applied research is concerned with applying current knowledge to real-world problems. This research aims to produce practical knowledge and solutions directly affecting real-world issues and circumstances (9).

This research type is undertaken to uncover solutions for issues relating to varying sectors like education, engineering, medicine, health, psychology, or business. Evaluation research, research and development, and action research are the types of applied research (10,11). Information is gathered using both quantitative and qualitative data collection techniques. For instance, a) Create a novel drug delivery system (NDDS) for cancer treatment with better therapeutic results and targeting efficiency. b) Research is required to determine whether a particular herb has therapeutic qualities.

d) **Fundamental research:** It is also known as basic or pure research. It is a type of scientific research to improve scientific theories and principles for better understanding and prediction of natural or other phenomena (12). E.g., a) Clarifying the genetic foundation of heredity in biology; b) Examining the role or underlying mechanisms of a recently identified protein target in the pathogenesis of Alzheimer's disease (AD). Although there may not be an apparent immediate use in this instance, the knowledge acquired adds to our understanding of neurodegenerative illnesses. It could guide future efforts to find drugs for AD and relatives' conditions.

e) **Quantitative research**: This strategy entails gathering and applying statistical techniques to numerical data analysis. It works well for studies that quantify variables and show how they relate. For instance, you may utilize quantitative techniques to assess a new drug's efficacy by analyzing how it affects biomarkers or patient symptoms (13).

f) **Qualitative research** aims to understand people's experiences, thoughts, and actions thoroughly. It entails gathering and numerically evaluating non-numerical data from sources like focus groups, observations, and interviews. Qualitative approaches help produce hypotheses and explore complex phenomena. For example, examining how patients feel about taking their medications as prescribed could assist in uncovering underlying causes and obstacles (14,15).

g) **Experimental research**: Empirical or experimental research focuses on changing factors and tracking how such changes affect results. It enables scientists to determine the causal linkages between various factors. Experiments are frequently employed in pharmaceutical research to evaluate the safety and effectiveness of novel medications or therapies. As an illustration, *a)* Carry out a randomized controlled experiment to evaluate the efficacy of two distinct therapies for a specific illness (16). *b)* The development of nanocarriers to target HIV-AIDS involves systematic experimentation aimed at developing effective and safe drug delivery systems (DDS).

h) **Conceptual research:** The fundamental definition of conceptual research is a methodology that involves monitoring and analyzing the current available information on a given issue. Although no actual experiments are conducted, it offers insightful information and recommendations for further study and real-world application (17)For instance, a conceptual framework that integrates essential ideas and tenets of personalized medicine can be used to direct clinical decision-making in oncology.

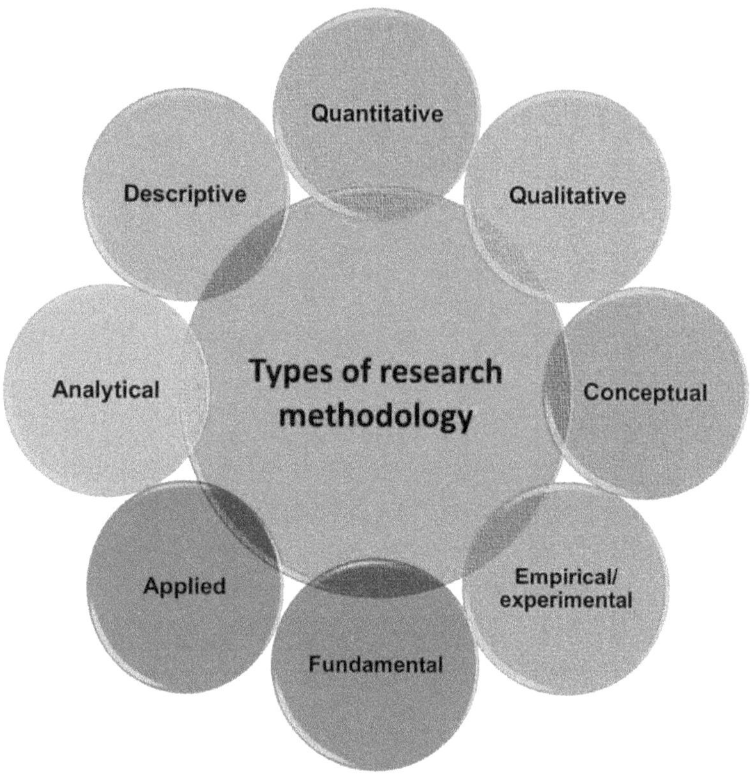

Image 4.1: Types of research methodology.

4.4 Experimental research

As was indicated in the previous section, pharmaceutical PhD programs across a range of areas mainly emphasize experimental research among all research approaches for several reasons (Image 4.2):

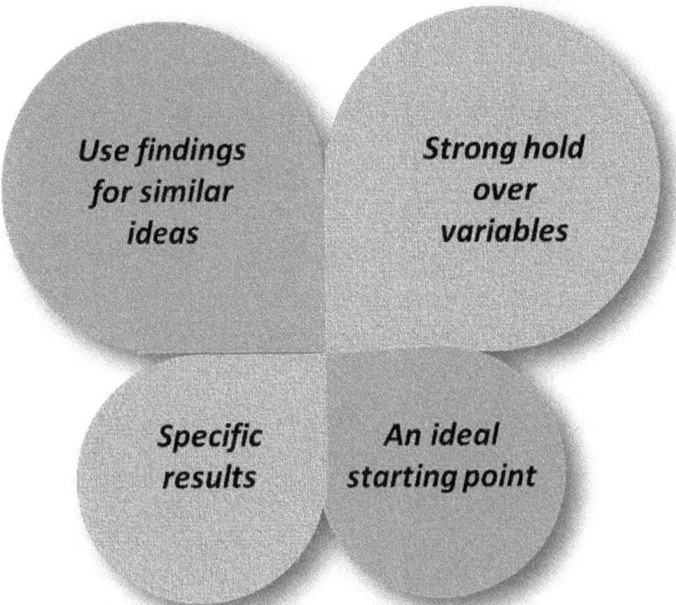

Image 4.2: Benefits of experimental research.

- **Advancing scientific knowledge:** This is the most objective and scientific approach. It enables PhD candidates to conduct research studies that further scientific understanding in their domains. The PhD students can test theories, produce new data, and advance knowledge of intricate pharmaceutical phenomena.

- **Problem-solving and innovation:** It covers issues and obstacles that arise in the pharmaceutical sciences in the actual world. It can create novel ideas, NDDS, and therapeutic strategies through experimenting to enhance healthcare results.

- **Hands-on training**: This research type teaches students essential laboratory techniques, experimental design, data analysis, and critical thinking skills, which are necessary for conducting

Independent research and pursuing careers in academia, industry, or government.

- **Validation of theories and models**: It enables candidates to corroborate or contradict pre-existing paradigms by validating ideas, models, and hypotheses.

- **Interdisciplinary collaboration**: It frequently entails multidisciplinary cooperation between scientists from different fields, including biology, chemistry, engineering, and medicine. The PhD candidates work together on cooperative research projects utilising various backgrounds and viewpoints to tackle complex pharmacological problems.

- **Translational research**: Translational research, which attempts to close the gap between fundamental scientific findings and therapeutic applications, is frequently the focus of experimental research. They conduct research to convert lab results into helpful remedies, cutting-edge medicines, and patient-beneficial medical procedures.

- **Publication and dissemination**: The results of experimental research are produced in data and discoveries that can be shared with the academic and professional world through patents, scientific publications, and conference presentations (18). Experimental research encompasses multiple stages, each of which we will discuss in detail in the following sections.

4.4.1   *Pre-formulation studies: An essential concept in formulation design*

Pre-formulation research is sometimes referred to as "Learning before doing." These are carried out to evaluate drug ingredients' chemical and physical characteristics before their preparation into dosage forms. To create safe, effective, and stable drug formulations, it is essential to comprehend the drug's intrinsic properties, such as solubility, stability, and compatibility with excipients. This research seeks to achieve this goal. Researchers can optimize formulation tactics, detect potential formulation issues, and guarantee the safety and efficacy of the final product by studying these qualities early in the development process (19).

i. **The primary objectives of pre-formulation studies**

- To produce the helpful data required to develop desired, convenient, stable,

  efficacious products at a large level.

- Before being developed into a final dosage form, establish a sophisticated understanding of the physicochemical properties (such as solubility, stability, and polymorphism) of novel pharmacological compounds (20).

- Assess the compatibility of drug substances with excipients and packaging materials.

- Identify potential degradation pathways and factors affecting drug stability.

- Optimize formulation parameters to enhance drug bioavailability and therapeutic efficacy.

- Provide essential data for selecting suitable formulation strategies and dosage forms (21,22).

ii. **Regulatory perspectives of pre-formulation studies**

Pre-formulation studies must adhere to several guidelines and pharmacopeial criteria to guarantee the efficacy, safety, and quality of pharmaceutical products. The standards and regulations that are frequently used are listed below.

a) **Indian Pharmacopoeia (IP), British Pharmacopoeia (BP), United States Pharmacopoeia (USP)**

An official compilation of recognized pharmaceutical standards is called the Pharmacopoeia. These standards offer requirements as well as testing protocols for dosage forms and pharmaceutical ingredients. Drug monographs, identification, purity, strength, quality attribute testing, and techniques for assessing medications' physical and chemical properties are typically included (23). As an example, for paracetamol in bulk and tablet formulations, the IP and BP both recommend titrimetric and UV spectrophotometric assay procedures (24).

b) **International council for harmonization of technical requirements for pharmaceuticals for human use (ICH)**

These recommendations offer standardized procedures and approaches for the creation of pharmaceuticals. ICH has progressively changed since its founding in 1990 to address the pharmaceutical industry's increasingly worldwide trends. An expanding number of regulatory bodies are also implementing these principles. Its goal is to increase global harmonization to guarantee that high-quality, safe, and effective medications are created, registered, and maintained in the most resource-efficient way possible while still upholding strict criteria (ich.org/). Q1A (R2) guidelines are used in pre-formulation analysis to examine pharmacological compounds under various stress scenarios. A coordinated attempt to standardize photostability testing on novel pharmaceutical compounds and products is the Q1B guideline. Quality risk management (QRM) utilizes the Q9 guideline.

c) **U.S. Food and Drug Administration guidelines (USFDA)**

The FDA guidelines include standards, recommendations, and regulatory requirements for the development of pharmaceuticals. Although there are no FDA standards for pre-formulation studies, many apply to different facets of pre-formulation research. For instance, the standards offer stability criteria and stress the use of quality by design (QbD) (25). Describe expectations for the characterization of drug compounds, including physicochemical properties, polymorphism, and impurity profiles, and offer suggestions for validating analytical procedures. The biopharmaceutics classification system (BCS), which classifies pharmacological compounds according to their permeability and solubility properties, is also included in this (26).

iii. Pre-formulation study challenges and mitigation

Table 4.1: Challenges and mitigation while conducting pre-formulation tests.

Challenges	Mitigation
Obtaining sufficient quantities of the drug substance for testing, especially in cases of limited availability or high cost.	Researchers should consider working with suppliers or investigating alternate synthesis pathways to guarantee a sufficient supply (27).
The complexity of analyzing physicochemical properties, such as solubility and stability, may require specialized equipment and expertise.	Collaborating with experienced analytical laboratories or utilizing advanced instrumentation can help address this challenge (28).
The reproducibility and reliability of results pose a challenge, mainly when dealing with sensitive or unstable compounds.	Implementing rigorous experimental protocols, conducting validation studies, and performing replicate analyses can help mitigate variability and enhance confidence in the data (29).
Navigating regulatory requirements and ensuring compliance can be challenging.	The regulatory approval process can be streamlined with careful documentation, adherence to set procedures, and

proactive communication with regulatory authorities.

(30).

By proactively addressing these problems and implementing appropriate mitigation mechanisms, researchers can successfully conduct pre-formulation investigations, which are crucial for pharmaceutical research and development.

iv. Parameters of pre-formulation studies

In pre-formulation evaluations, several key parameters are considered to comprehensively assess the characteristics of drug substances.

Physicochemical characterization

a) *Physical parameters*

Organoleptic properties

The first step in pre-formulation is a thorough explanation of the organoleptic characteristics of the drug compounds, such as color, flavor, texture, and taste (31,32). These are mentioned briefly in following Table 4.2.

Table 4.2: Organoleptic properties of drug substances.

Parameters	Significance	Techniques
Colour	Indication of purity, identity, and stability.	Colourimetry, spectrophotometry, and visual inspection.
Odour	Examine any contamination, deterioration of the chemical composition, or volatile component presence.	Olfactometry, gas chromatography-mass spectrometry (GC-MS), and electronic nose (e-nose) devices.
Appearance	Assist in locating flaws, extraneous	Visual inspection, microscopy, and imaging

	objects, and modifications to physical characteristics.	techniques (e.g., scanning electron microscopy, optical microscopy.
Texture	It includes hardness, smoothness, grittiness, and stickiness. It affects product handling, administration, and overall sensory experience.	Texture analyzer (31,32).

b) *Chemical parameters*

Table 4.3: Chemical properties of drug substances.

Parameters	Significance	Techniques
Melting Point	Examine the chemical's crystalline structure and other physical characteristics. Generally, impurities increase and lower the melting point's range.	Differential scanning calorimetry (DSC), capillary tube method, and melting point apparatus (33).
Solubility	Understanding a drug's ability to dissolve in various solvents aids in optimizing formulation composition, dosage forms, and DDS to enhance drug absorption and bioavailability.	UV-visible spectroscopy, shake-flask method, gravimetric analysis, and titration (22,34).
pH	It evaluates the alkalinity or acidity of	Benchtop pH meters (35).

	medicinal ingredients and formulations. This affects the effectiveness and safety of pharmaceutical products, their solubility, compatibility with excipients, and stability.	
Partition coefficient (log P)	Estimating a compound's lipophilicity and membrane permeability. It is a predictive method that affects medication bioavailability and pharmacokinetics by predicting drug absorption, distribution, metabolism, and excretion (ADME).	Chromatographic technique, computational model, liquid-liquid extraction (36).
Polymorphism	The ability of a substance to exist in multiple crystalline forms or structures influences its physical and chemical properties. This plays a crucial role in drug development, affecting drug stability, solubility, bioavailability, and formulation design.	X-ray powder diffraction (XRPD), DSC (37).
Hygroscopicity	A material's capacity to absorb moisture from its surroundings affects its	Dynamic vapor sorption (DVS), gravimetric moisture

processing, stability, and effectiveness in medicine formulations. This ensures pharmaceutical medicines' effectiveness, safety, and quality, especially those prone to moisture deterioration.	sorption analysis (GMSA), Karl Fischer titration (38,39).

c) *Solid-state characterization*

Flow properties

The qualities of a material that control how it behaves in the presence of outside forces, like gravity or mechanical agitation, are referred to as flow properties. It provides essential information about the properties of the powder, including the size, shape, and density of the particles. Numerous factors, including the angle of repose (AOR), Carr's index, bulk density (Pb), tapped density (Pt), etc., can be used to estimate it (40).

Table 4.4: Flow properties of the drug.

Pre-formulation test name	Formula	Observations	Properties
The angle of repose (flow behaviour of granule)	$AOR = Tan\theta^{-1}(2h/d)$	<20	Excellent flow
		20–30	Free-flowing
		30–34	Passable flow
		>40	Poor flow (41).

Bulk density (individual particle arrangement)	$Pb = M/Vo$	> 0.5 g/ml (high value)	Limitation to flow
Tapped density (degree of powder packing, cohesiveness)	$Pt = M/Vt$	High density	Better flow (42).
Inter-particle porosity (Ie) (void space between particles)	$Ie = \{(Pb - Pt)/(Pb \times Pt)\}$	-	(43).
Carr Index (CI%, strength, stability, and compressibility)	$CI = ((Pb - Pt)/Pt)$	<0.10	Excellent flow
		0.26–0.31	Poor flow (44).
Hausner ratio (HR, inter-particulate friction, and compressibility)	$HR = Pt/Pb$	1.00–1.11	Free-flowing
		1.35–1.45	Poor flow (20).

Vo: volume, M: known weight, Vt: tapped volume in measuring cylinder, Pb: bulk density, Pt: tapped density, AOR: angle of repose; h: heap height, d: horizontal base diameter.

d)   Particle Size Determination (PSD)

The method of determining the size of particles in a sample is known as particle size analysis. Particle size is vital in pharmaceuticals for:

- Controlling drug dissolution rates, which impacts bioavailability and onset of action.
- Ensuring uniformity and stability of drug formulations.
- Enhancing DDS for targeted and controlled release.
- Improving process efficiency during manufacturing (45).

Particle size can affect essential metrics include surface area and crystallinity. Although they are frequently assessed in conjunction with particle size to offer more information about the physical characteristics of the particles, they are not usually utilized directly for PSD. The total area of all the particle surfaces in a specific volume of material is called the **surface area.** Particle surface area increases as particle size decreases. It impacts how rapidly medications dissolve and interact with other bodily chemicals. The arrangement of atoms within a substance is referred to as **crystallinity**. It modifies the stability, solubility, and other characteristics of the medication.

Table 4.5: Techniques used to determine particle size.

Particle size determination

Techniques	Significance
Microscopy: 1. Optical microscopy 2. Scanning electron microscopy (SEM) 3. Transmission electron microscopy (TEM) 4. Hot stage microscopy	• Provide visual data on particle size and morphology (46). • This technique magnifies the sample and scans it with electrons, producing detailed images that help determine particle sizes (47). • Similar to SEM but provides even higher resolution images, suitable for analyzing very small particles (48). • Observes particles under a microscope while heating them gradually, which helps understand how particle sizes change with temperature (49).
Laser diffraction	Measures the scattering pattern of laser light passing through a sample to determine particle size distribution (50).
Dynamic light scattering (DLS)	Analyse fluctuations in scattered light intensity to determine PSD in suspensions or colloidal systems (51).

Sieve analysis	Uses a series of sieves with progressively smaller openings to separate particles based on size (52).
Coulter counter	Measures change in electrical impedance as particles pass through a small orifice, providing information on particle size distribution (53).
Sedimentation method	It utilizes the rate at which particles settle under the influence of gravity in a liquid medium to determine PSD (54).
Particles surface area	
Brunauer-Emmett-Teller (BET) method	Measures surface area by analyzing the adsorption of gas molecules onto the surface of particles (55).
Gas adsorption techniques	Utilizes the adsorption of gas molecules onto the surface of particles to calculate surface area (56).
Crystallinity	
XRD	Determines a material's crystal structure and phase composition by analyzing how X-rays are diffracted by its atoms (57).
DSC	Detects changes in heat flow associated with crystalline transitions like melting or recrystallization, providing insights into the material's crystallinity (58).

e)   Analytical characterization

Analytical characterisation can identify, isolate, and quantify chemicals and materials or describe their physical properties. Measuring variables such as retention time, peak area, absorbance, and crystalline index provides crucial details regarding composition, structure, and attributes (59). It includes various analytical techniques, such as spectroscopy, chromatography, and gravimetry.

Objectives:

- Identify and quantify the active pharmaceutical ingredient (API) in a drug formulation.
- To assess the purity, stability, and degradation of API products.
- To characterize the physical properties of the API, such as particle size, shape, and surface area.
- To investigate the compatibility of the API with excipients and packaging materials.
- To establish analytical methods for quality control and stability testing of drug products.

Techniques	**Summary**
UV-visible spectroscopy	**Determination of absorption maxima** Absorption maxima, represented by λmax, indicate the wavelength at which a substance absorbs light most strongly (60). **Preparation of standard calibration curve** Essential for quantifying the concentration of a substance in a sample. It provides a relationship between concentration and the response of the analytical instrument. $y = mx + b$ y - the instrument response x - the concentration of the analyte m- the slope, and b - the y-intercept (61).
Fourier transform infrared spectroscopy (FTIR)	It is a powerful technique for analyzing the functional groups and chemical bonds present in a sample by measuring the absorption of infrared radiation (62).
Differential scanning calorimetry	DSC is a thermal analysis technique used to study the thermal behaviour of materials, including phase transitions, melting points, and heat capacities. Changes in heat flow, such as endothermic or

	Exothermic peaks provide information about the sample's thermal properties (63). This is essential in pharmaceutical research for characterizing drug polymorphism, stability, and compatibility (64).
X-ray Diffraction	An approach for examining a material's crystalline structure. It's essential for determining and describing salts, crystallinity, and drug polymorphs (57).
Mass spectroscopy	It aids in identifying and quantifying the molecular composition of compounds within a sample by ionizing molecules and separating them based on their mass-to-charge ratio (65).
High-performance liquid chromatography (HPLC)	It is essential for assessing drug and excipient compatibility in pharmaceutical research. It separates and quantifies individual components within complex samples, like pharmaceutical formulations, enabling precise identification and quantification of various compounds (66).
Thermogravimetric analysis (TGA)	It measures the drug molecule's mass change as a function of temperature. It helps assess thermal stability, moisture content, and volatile component loss.

Table 4.6: Common analytical techniques.

f)   Stability study

Something is said to be stable if it remains constant across time. Stability in the context of pharmaceuticals refers to a product's quality continuing to be constant throughout its manufacturing process without any changes to its features or attributes. Stability is generally determined by five key factors: chemical, physical, therapeutic, microbiological, and toxicological (67). It is used to determine the effects of environmental conditions on product quality.

Importance of stability studies

- Because the active drug's dose form lowers as it becomes unstable, undermedication may result.

- Toxic products may result from the medicine or product's breakdown.

- The medication can alter its physical characteristics when being marketed from one location to another while transported.

- One possible cause of instability could be a physical appearance change. Drug stability is predicted using kinetics concepts; however, kinetics and stability studies are not the same (68).

Table 4.7: Codes and titles used in ICH guidelines.

ICH code	Guideline title
Q1A	Stability testing of new drug substances and products (second revision)
Q1B	Stability testing: Photostability testing of new drug substances and products
Q1C	Stability testing of new dosage forms
Q1D	Bracketing and matrixing designs for stability testing of drug substances and products
Q1E	Evaluation of stability data
Q1F	Stability data package for registration applications in climatic zones III and IV
Q5C	Stability testing of biotechnological/biological products (69).

Table 4.8: Types of stability studies (ICH Q1A (R2).

Study type	Storage condition	Minimum time period covered by data at submission

Long term	25 °C ± 2 °C/60% RH ± 5% RH or at 30 °C ± 2 °C/65% RH ± 5% RH	12 months
Intermediate	30°C ± 2°C/65% RH ± 5% RH	6 months
Accelerated	40 °C ± 2 °C/75% RH ± 5% RH	6 months (70,71).

RH: Relative humidity.

4.4.2 *Preliminary analysis of pharmacogenetic plants*

Pharmacogenetic evaluation helps to screen commercial varieties, substitutes, adulterants, and any other quality control of herbal drugs. It is a simple and reliable tool that helps to obtain information about the biochemical and physical properties of herbs (72). Preliminary screening includes quality control tests, extraction, phytochemical evaluation, and identification. The following section briefly discusses each step.

i. *Quality control test*

Quality control tests such as loss on drying (LOD), ash value, and extractive value measurements serve as fundamental benchmarks for assessing the purity and consistency of herbal materials. These tests provide insights into the presence of impurities, moisture content, and overall quality of the botanicals under scrutiny (73).

These are done for several purposes:

- Assessment of purity
- Detection of adulteration
- Evaluation of stability
- Standardization of products
- Assurance of safety.

Table 4.9: Quality control test along with the significance.

Test name	Significance
Loss on drying	The stability and purity of the material determine the moisture content, which can affect the quality and shelf life of the product.
Ash value	It indicates the amount of inorganic material present, which can help assess the purity of the material and detect the presence of adulterants (74).
Extractive value	It provides information about the solubility of active constituents in the sample, which is essential for assessing the material's potential efficacy.

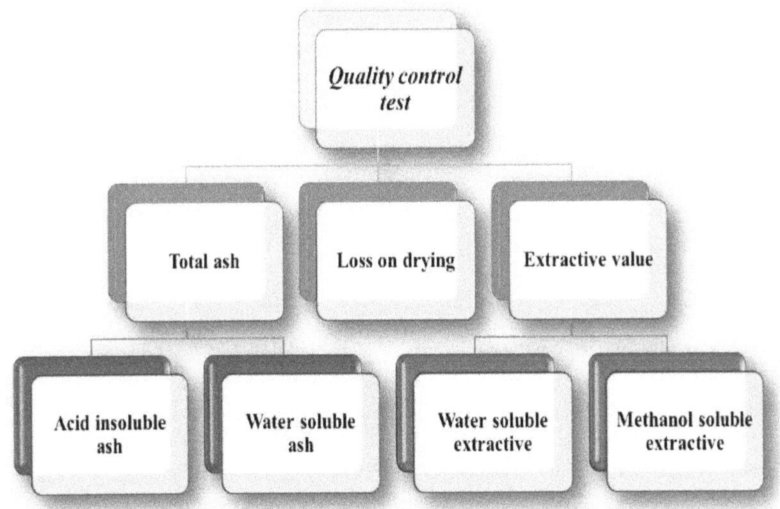

Image 4.3: Parameters of quality control test.

Formula to calculate quality control tests

1. Loss on drying (LOD):

$$LOD\ (\%) = \frac{Initial\ weight\ of\ sample - Weight\ of\ sample\ after\ Drying}{Initial\ weight\ of\ sampl} x\ 100$$

2. Ash value:

$$Ash\ Value(\%) = \frac{Weight\ of\ ash}{Weight\ of\ sample} X\ 100$$

3. Extractive value:

$$Extractive\ Value(\%) = \frac{Weight\ of\ extract}{Weight\ of\ Sample} x\ 100$$

ii.   *Preliminary phytochemical studies*

Phytochemical screening is the initial step in preserving the quality of plants or herbal extracts. It helps distinguish between the constituents of extracts and those that predominate over the others. However, it also helps search for bioactive compounds that can be employed to make necessary pharmaceuticals. It entails several procedures meant to detect distinct chemical components in plant extracts. Alkaloids, sugars, flavonoids, saponins, and other types of chemicals are frequently evaluated in these studies. These offer insightful information about the chemical makeup of plant extracts and set the stage for future research into their possible therapeutic uses (75).

Table 4.10: Preliminary phytochemical tests (76–79).

Test	Observations
Detection of alkaloids	
Dragendroff's/ Kraut's test	A reddish-brown precipitate (ppt)
Hager's test	A creamy white ppt
Mayer's/ Bertrand's/ Valser's test	A creamy white/yellow ppt
Wagner's test	A brown/reddish ppt
Picric acid test	orange colour
Iodine Test	A blue colour
Bouchardat's test	A reddish-brown colour
Tannic acid test	A buff colour ppt

Detection of carbohydrates

Barfoed's test	A red ppt
Molisch test	A violet ring
Seliwanoff's Test	A rose-red colour {ketoses}
Resorcinol test	A rose colour {ketones}
Test for pentoses	A red colour
Test for starch	A binary colouration
Reducing sugars	
Benedict's test	Green/yellow/red colour
Fehling's test	A red ppt

Detection of glycosides

Borntrager's test	A pink coloured solution
Modified Borntrager's test	A rose-pink to blood-red coloured solution
Legal's test	A pink coloured solution
10% NaOH test	A brick-red ppt
Aqueous NaOH test	A yellow colour
Conc. H_2SO_4 test	A brown ring
Raymond's test	A violet colour
Keller-Killani test	A blue-coloured solution (in an acetic acid layer)
Kedee's test	A disappearing violet colour
Bromine water test	A yellow precipitate
Baljet test	A yellow-orange colour

Detection of proteins and amino acids

Biuret test	A pink-coloured sol.
Millon's test	A white ppt
Ninhydrin test	A purple-coloured sol. {Amino acids}
Xanthoproteic test	A yellow-coloured sol.

Detection of flavonoids

Alkaline reagent test	An intense yellow colour becomes colourless with the addition of diluted acid.
Lead acetate test	A yellow fluorescence
Shinoda's test	A yellow ppt
Shibata's reaction/	A pink to crimson coloured solution

Cyanidin test	
Ferric chloride test	A green ppt
Ammonia test	A yellow colour
Conc. H$_2$SO4 test	An orange colour

Detection of phenolic compounds

Iodine test	A transient red colour
Ferric chloride test	Dark green/bluish-black colour
Gelatin test	A white precipitate
Lead acetate test	A white precipitate
Ellagic Acid Test	The solution turns muddy /Niger brown precipitate
Potassium dichromate test	A dark colour
Hot water test	Black or brown colour ring at the junction of dipping
Test for Carotenoids	A blue colour at the interface

Detection of tannins

Gelatin test	A white precipitate
Braymer's test	Blue-green colour
10% NaOH test	Formation of emulsion {Hydrolysable tannins}
Bromine water test	Decolouration of bromine
Lead subacetate test	A creamy gelatinous ppt
Phenazone test	Precipitation
Mitchell's test	A water-soluble iron-tannin complex, which is insoluble in a solution of ammonium acetate
HCl test	A red precipitate
Foam test	Formation of a 2 cm thick layer of foam
NaHCO$_3$ test	Stable honeycomb-like froth
Olive oil test	Appearance of foam
Haemolysis test	Zone of haemolysis

Detection of phytosterols

Salkowski's test	Red colour

Libermann-Burchard's test	An array of colour change
Acetic anhydride test	Change in colour from violet to blue/green
Hesse's response	Pink ring / Red colour
Sulphur test	Sulphur sinks to the bottom
Detection of Cholesterol	A red-rose colour
Detection of Terpenoids	A grey-coloured solution

Detection of triterpenoids

Salkowski's test	Golden yellow layer
Diterpenes-Copper acetate test	Emerald green colour
Lignins-Furfuraldehyde test	A red colour
Carotenoids-Carr-Price reaction	A blue-green colour, eventually changing to red

Detection of quinones

Alcoholic KOH test	Red to blue colour
Conc. HCl test	A green colour
Sulphuric acid test	A red colour

Detection of anthraquinones

Borntrager's test	A pink, violet, or red coloured solution
Ammonium hydroxide test	Formation of red colour after 2 min.

Detection of anthocyanins

HCl test	Pink-red sol. which turns blue-violet after addition of ammonia
Leuconthocyanins Isoamyl alcohol test	The upper layer appears red
Carboxylic acid Effervescence test	Appearance of Effervescence

Detection of coumarins

NaOH paper test	Yellow fluorescence under UV light
NaOH test	A yellow colour

Detection of Emodin	A red colour
Gums and Mucilage Alcohol test	A white or cloudy precipitate

Detection of resins

Acetic anhydride test	Orange to yellow
Turbidity test	Turbidity

Detection of fixed oils and fat/ volatile oil

Spot test/ Stain test	Oil stain on the paper
Saponification test	Soap formation or partial alkali neutralisation
Fluorescence test	Bright pinkish fluorescence

iii.   *Identification of phytoconstituents*

Plant extracts contain various bioactive chemicals with different polarities, making identifying and characterising and challenging. It is normal to recognize and separate these bioactive chemicals utilizing separation procedures to obtain pure molecules. Plant chemical components are identified using IR, GC-MS, and UV-vis spectroscopy; the mixtures are separated and analyzed using TLC and HPLC (80). By comparing the results obtained from these techniques with known standards or reference data, researchers can accurately identify phytoconstituents present in their samples (81).

4.4.3   Role of artificial intelligence in pre-formulation studies

a) **Data analysis and prediction:** Large volumes of data from many sources, including research articles, chemical databases, and experimental results, can be analyzed by AI algorithms to find trends and patterns that are pertinent to pre-formulation investigations (82).

b) **Formulation optimization:** AI models can optimize formulation parameters such as excipient selection, drug dosage, and delivery systems by simulating and predicting their effects on drug stability, solubility, and bioavailability (20).

c) **Virtual screening:** During the early phases of drug development, time and resources can be saved by using AI-based virtual screening techniques to effectively discover possible drug candidates or excipients by anticipating their physicochemical features, interactions, and suitability for particular formulations (83).

d) **Drug-excipient compatibility prediction:** To anticipate whether medicinal ingredients and excipients would be compatible, artificial intelligence (AI) models can examine molecular structures and properties. This helps prevent formulation problems such as drug degradation or instability (84).

e) **Process optimization:** By evaluating data from formulation tests and process factors, artificial intelligence (AI) may optimize industrial processes to improve product quality, lower costs, and shorten production times (85,86).

f) **Quality control:** AI-based systems can monitor and analyze real-time data during manufacturing processes to detect deviations from desired specifications, ensuring the quality and consistency of pharmaceutical products (87).

g) **Decision support:** By offering insights, suggestions, and forecasts based on intricate data analysis, artificial intelligence (AI) tools can help researchers and formulators make well-informed decisions, which will ultimately result in more successful and efficient pre-formulation studies (88).

4.5 Drug excipients compatibility studies

4.5.1 Overview of DECS

To guarantee the stability, safety, and effectiveness of pharmaceutical products, pharmaceuticals, and excipients must be compatible. Inactive substances called excipients are added to medications to help with production, administration, and efficacy. However, the final formulation's chemical, physical, and biological properties may be impacted by interactions between medications and excipients (89). Thus, understanding and assessing the compatibility between drugs and excipients is essential to prevent undesirable outcomes such as degradation, reduced efficacy, or adverse patient reactions. To assess these interactions, compatibility studies include a variety of analytical techniques and procedures, from eye inspection to complex spectroscopic and chromatographic tests. In pharmaceutical research and development, comprehensive analysis and evaluation of DECS are essential phases that direct the creation and refinement of potent and stable medicinal formulations.

Techniques to determine DECS

a) Visual inspection

It entails examining the mixture's outward features, including its color, texture, and smell. Variations in these areas may be a sign of impending issues. For instance, if the color shifts or intensifies, this could indicate degradation or chemical interactions. Likewise, clumps or strange textures may indicate compatibility or mixing problems (90). Strong or unusual odours may also be signs of volatile compound releases or chemical reactions. Visual inspection provides important qualitative information regarding the formulation's appearance and cohesiveness. It aids in the early detection of possible problems so that we can use more sophisticated methods to look into them further. By watching for these visual cues, researchers can ensure that pharmaceutical formulations are optimized for stability, effectiveness, and safety (22).

b)   ***Analytical techniques to evaluate DECS***

- Fourier transform infrared spectroscopy
- Differential scanning calorimetry
- X-ray diffraction study
- Microscopic techniques (SEM, TEM)
- UV-Vis spectroscopy
- High-Performance Liquid Chromatography
- Mass spectroscopy
- Nuclear Magnetic Resonance spectroscopy (*see above section for more details)*
- Raman spectroscopy

Raman spectroscopy uses the inelastic scattering of monochromatic light to provide fine-grained molecular insights into composition and interactions. Chemical structure changes can be found thanks to this method and its sensitivity to minute variations in molecule vibrations (91). Using this approach, researchers can find possible interactions, intricate forms, or degradation processes that might affect a formulation's stability or effectiveness. It is beneficial for researching polymorphic transitions and crystalline structures, which helps comprehend solid-state alterations that are essential for formulation performance. Because of its non-destructive qualities and adaptability, it is invaluable for continuous quality control and monitoring during the formulation process, enabling well-informed choices and pharmaceutical product optimisations (92).

4.6 Formulation and optimization of trial batches

Any dosage form formulation necessitates following set protocols. To guarantee the effectiveness of this stage, a thorough assessment of the literature is necessary. Depending on the physicochemical characteristics, the dosage form being developed, the manufacturing scale, the regulations, etc., it involves different methods and techniques. (93) For example, the Extrusion-Spheronization method forms spherical pellets or beads used in controlled-release dosage forms. The method commonly used to develop dendrimers is known as the "Divergent growth approach" (94). The solvent casting method is utilized for transdermal patch preparation. To put it briefly, there are several ways to formulate dosage forms, and the approach that is chosen relies on a number of variables, including the researcher's preferences, the resources at hand, the goals of the study, and the particulars of the formulation that is being developed. As is well known, trial batches of the formulation must be prepared to ensure validity and dependability; depending only on the outcomes of a single batch is insufficient. The primary goal of preparing trial batches is to evaluate and contrast various formulations. In addition, it has several benefits for regulatory compliance, market testing, process improvement, optimization, risk mitigation, quality assurance, and confidence-building (95). Through meticulous testing and analysis, trial batches aid in crafting medications that deliver maximum therapeutic benefits. In the world of medicine, finding the best way to make medicines work well is important. This involves trying out different forms of medicine, like pills or syrups. A significant portion of this involves creating the right number of test batches using the right techniques. These trial batches aid scientists determine the most effective medication production method. They also assist in determining the optimal dosage form for a given combination of substances. Through meticulous testing and analysis of the outcomes, this approach aids scientists in creating medications that are effective for patients (96).

4.6.1   *Optimization of trial batches*

Optimizing means making something ideal, practical, or as functional as feasible. It determines the most effective use of available resources while considering all the factors influencing decision-making in any experiment. OR it is the process of improving something or making it work better. Optimization has always meant changing one variable at a time to solve a problem formulation in the pharmaceutical industry. To improve formulation irregularities, the design of experiments (DoE) (97) Is used. Its importance stems from its capacity to methodically investigate many elements and their combinations to identify the ideal circumstances or configurations for a given procedure or output (98).

4.6.2   *Why is an optimization so important?*

Take on the role of a cake baker. It should be just the appropriate amount of sweetness, not too dry, and have the ideal texture. You might try experimenting with different amounts of flour, sugar, eggs, and baking time until you find the ideal blend to do this. Likewise, optimization plays a vital part in research and industry when it comes to creating new medicine formulations or streamlining manufacturing processes. Think of it like a cake that tastes just the way you want it to (99).

Having a clever plan for the experimenting process is similar to the design of experiments. DOE methodically assists in planning experiments instead of haphazardly altering variables and hoping for the best results. It analyzes the effects of many parameters on your result, including temperature, duration, composition or pH, and excipient ratios. Because it helps you focus on what is actually important and prevent needless trial and error, this strategy helps you save time and resources (100).

4.6.3   *Benefits of optimization*

a) **Enhanced efficacy**: Optimization allows for the refinement of drug formulations to maximize therapeutic effectiveness, ensuring that the medication achieves its intended clinical outcomes (101).

b) **Improved safety profile:** Optimization helps minimize possible side effects by fine-tuning dosage schedules and formulations, improving the drug's patient safety profile.

c) **Cost efficiency**: Optimizing drug development processes reduces resource wastage by streamlining experimentation and manufacturing processes, leading to significant cost savings over time (102).

d) **Accelerated development timelines**: Through systematic optimization, drug development timelines can be expedited, allowing promising candidates to reach the market faster and address unmet medical needs sooner.

e) **Tailored patient treatment**: Optimization makes it easier to tailor medication formulations to the unique requirements of patient groups, taking into account elements like dosage form, frequency of dosing, and administration method.

f) **Increased drug stability**: Optimization efforts can improve the stability and shelf-life of pharmaceutical products, ensuring their integrity and efficacy throughout storage and distribution (103).

g) **Regulatory compliance:** Improved medication development procedures follow regulations more precisely, lowering the possibility of roadblocks and speeding up approval procedures.

4.6.4 Methods of optimization
Factorial Designs:

In the 1800s, Joseph Henry Gilbert and John Bennet Lawes were the first to use factorial designs (FD). Most of these are derived from mathematical models of the first order. First, while considering treatment modifications, candidates always choose FD. Contrarily, factorial designs are successful. Combining this research into one would be more efficient than conducting several separate studies. FD types include:

- Fractional factorial design
- Star design
- Plackett-Burman designs (97).

Let's examine a fictitious clinical trial that aims to determine whether a novel medication effectively treats hypertension. The researchers wish to examine two parameters: dosage and administration duration.

Factor 1: Dosage

- Level 1: Low dosage (50 mg)
- Level 2: High dosage (100 mg)

Factor 2: Administration time

- Level 1: Morning administration
- Level 2: Evening administration

Patients participating in the study would be randomly assigned to one of the four treatment groups:

1. Low dosage in the morning
2. Low dosage in the evening
3. High dosage in the morning
4. High dosage in the evening

Table 4.11: 2 x 2 factorial design.

		Administration time	
		Morning	Evening
Dosage	Low dose	Low dosage in the morning	Low dosage in the evening
	High dose	High dosage in the morning	High dosage in the evening

The allocated therapy would be administered to each group for a predetermined amount of time, and the outcome variable after the experiment would be the researchers' measurement of the drop in blood pressure. Researchers can therefore evaluate the effects of administration duration and dosage, as well as any potential interactions between the two elements, by utilizing a 2x2 factorial design.

This design allows for efficient evaluation of multiple factors simultaneously and provides insights into their individual and combined effects on the outcome of interest.

Response surface methodology (RSM):

It is a mathematical and statistical method that is frequently applied in DoE. The response variable of interest and the independent variables that affect it are the focus of the response variable optimization and understanding process (RSM) (104). They are helpful when the linear functions cannot be applied (105). Creating an empirical model that explains the response variable's behaviour inside the experimental domain is the response surface methodology's primary (RSM) objective. A second-order polynomial that connects the response variable to the independent variables is commonly used to illustrate this model. The purpose of these well-planned experiments is to effectively explore the factor space, maximising the amount of information obtained while minimizing the number of tests needed. Model parameters are estimated using regression analysis after the experimental data are gathered. The estimated model can determine ideal settings, comprehend the relationship between causes and responses, and forecast response variables under various circumstances. The technique is frequently used to optimize studies in a variety of sectors, including chemical, mechanical, biological, environmental, and pharmaceutical because it is simple to understand and involves little experimentation (106,107). *Box-Behnken* (108) *Central composite,* (109) *and Doehlert designs* are the type of RSM.

a) **3D plots**: 3D plots represent the response surface in three dimensions in RSM. Each axis typically represents one of the independent variables, and the response value is plotted on the z-axis. This allows you to visualize how the response changes as you move through the space defined by the independent variables.

b) **Contour plots**: Contour plots are two-dimensional graphical depictions of the response surface. Curves depicting the behavior of the response surface are created by connecting points with the same response value using lines or contours. The form of the surface may be seen, and regions of interest, such as areas of maximum or minimum response, can be found using contour plots (110).

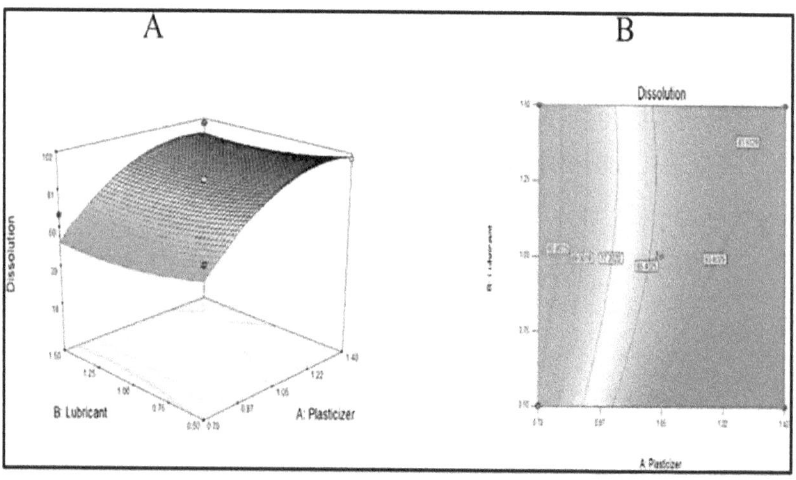

Image 4.4: 3D and Countor plots describe the impact of lubricant and plasticizer on drug Release (111).

4.7   Evaluation of prepared formulation/ dosage form

The word **"dosage forms"** describes pharmaceutical preparations or formulations designed to make administering and delivering active pharmaceutical substances more accessible and more precisely. These formulations consist of a particular blend of drug substances (API) and inert components (excipients). Evaluating a dosage form's chemical, biological, and physical characteristics is part of its characterization. This procedure is essential to the research and production of pharmaceuticals to ensure that the dosage form delivers the API precisely, reliably, and effectively. Based on their physical states, dosage forms are often divided into three categories in pharmaceutical development and manufacturing: semisolid, solid, and liquid. Before being authorized for clinical use, every kind of dosage form is subjected to extensive assessment.

Importance of evaluation of dosage form

- Safety assurance
- Quality control
- Consistency
- Regulatory compliance
- Effectiveness
- Identifying impurities
- Optimization of formulation
- Long-term stability quality assurance
- Customer trust (51).

To determine their appearance, texture, and consistency, several parameters are used to evaluate semisolid dosage forms, such as creams, ointments, gels, and pastes (111). Solid dosage forms encompass tablets, capsules, powders, granules, suppositories, and lozenges. These formulations consist primarily of solid particles and are intended for oral administration (112). Liquid dosage forms include solutions, suspensions, emulsions, syrups, and elixirs. These formulations are characterized by their fluid consistency and are suitable for oral, topical, or parenteral administration (113). Evaluation of dosage form includes the following parameters (Image 4.5).

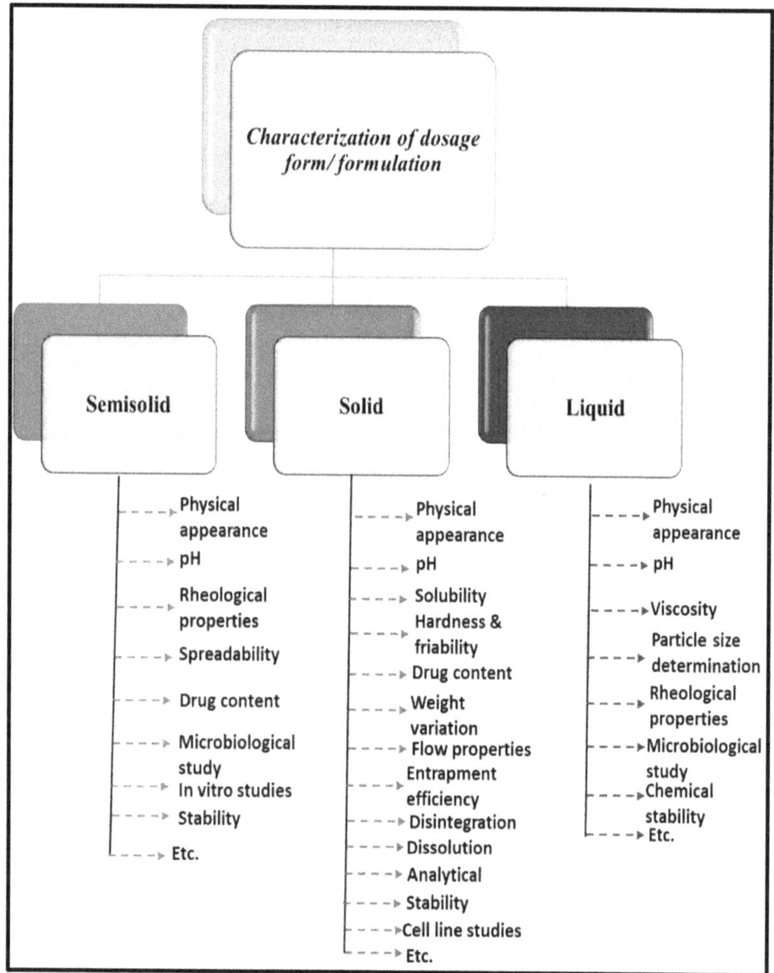

Image 4.5: Evaluation parameters of the dosage form.

4.7.1   Physical Appearance and pH Determination

Physical appearance assessment involves observing colour, texture, uniformity, and the presence of any defects or foreign particles in dosage form (114). While pH measurement is crucial for formulations intended for topical or mucosal administration as it affects skin irritation potential and stability.

4.7.2   Viscosity

Viscosity affects semisolid dosage forms' consistency, spreadability, and flow behavior, affecting how easy and stable they are to apply. It is also determinable for the compositions in liquid form. Viscosity is measured using rheometers or viscometers (115).

4.7.3   Spreadability

Their spreadability measures the ability of semisolid dosage forms to disperse uniformly across a surface. Patient convenience and compliance can be improved by applying and distributing a formulation with good spread ability across the application area. Good spreadability helps the active components penetrate the skin more deeply, increasing their bioavailability and therapeutic benefits. It can be assessed with tools such as the Burett or Gillissen methods (116).

$$S = \frac{M}{L} X\, T$$

Where S= Spreadability, M = Weight in the pan L = Length of a glass slide and T = Time (in sec.) taken to separate the slides (117).

4.7.4   Drug content uniformity

Assuring that the active ingredient's concentration remains constant throughout the formulation is known as "drug content uniformity." This is necessary to guarantee the patient receives the prescribed medication dosage each time. Drug efficacy and safety may be compromised by under- or overdose as a result of inaccurate drug content. Consistency in the amount of medication provided to the patient is ensured by maintaining a homogeneous drug content throughout the formulation, which results in consistent therapeutic effects. Methods: titration, UV-visible spectroscopy, HPLC, etc (118).

4.7.5   Hardness and friability

Hardness indicates the resistance of solid dosage forms to mechanical stress during handling and transportation, while friability assesses their tendency to crumble or break apart. It ensures the tablet's strength and integrity, which are vital for manufacturing, packaging, and patient use (119). A hardness tester is used for hardness testing, while a friability tester is employed to determine friability.

4.7.6   Weight variation

It evaluates how consistently dose units, like tablets or capsules, are distributed throughout a batch of solid dosage forms. It assures that the right amount of active substance is present in every unit, resulting in constant patient dosage. It entails weighing each dose unit and comparing the weights to the acceptance standards (or guidelines) defined in regulatory guidelines or pharmacopeial standards (120). The technique used is precision balance or analytical balance.

4.7.7   Flow properties

The manufacturability of solid dosage forms is impacted by flow characteristics, which impact procedures including filling, compression, and blending. In production, homogeneity and reproducibility are ensured by proper flow (*See above section*).

4.7.8   Entrapment efficiency

Entrapment efficiency is crucial in solid dosage form development, particularly for formulations involving drug encapsulation or entrapment within carriers like nanoparticles or microspheres. It measures the proportion of the drug successfully trapped or encapsulated within the carrier, indicating the formulation's effectiveness in delivering the intended dose.

Techniques: Ultracentrifugation, filtration, or dialysis combined with analytical methods are used to analyze the concentration of drug within the carrier matrix, allowing calculation of the entrapped efficiency (121).

$$Entrapment\ efficiency\ (\%) = \frac{Amount\ of\ drug\ entrapped}{Total\ amount\ of\ drug\ added}\ X\ 100$$

4.7.9   Loading capacity

It assesses the maximum amount of drug that can be incorporated into a carrier matrix in solid dosage forms, such as nanoparticles or microspheres. This is important because it determines the maximum dosage strength achievable and influences the formulation's efficacy and performance. Techniques: Spectrophotometer or HPLC (122).

$$Loading\ capacity = \frac{Amount\ of\ drug\ entrapped}{Weight\ of\ carrier}\ X\ 100$$

4.7.10   Disintegration

Disintegration is necessary for solid dose forms like tablets and capsules to dissolve swiftly and eventually in the gastrointestinal tract. It evaluates the dosage form's capacity to break down into smaller pieces so the body can release and absorb the medication more effectively. Methods: USP Disintegration Device (123).

4.7.11   Dissolution

Dissolution assesses the rate and extent of drug release from solid dosage forms. It provides valuable information on how the dosage form behaves in simulated physiological conditions, indicating its effectiveness in delivering the drug to the body. Techniques: Dissolution tester or dissolution apparatus (paddle, basket, or flow-through apparatus) (125).

4.7.12   Solubility

Determining the dissolving behavior and formulation viability of poorly soluble medicines is essential for influencing drug absorption and bioavailability (34).

4.7.13   Particle size determination

Particle size influences drug dissolution rate, absorption, stability, and formulation performance. It is particularly for solid dosage forms and particulate delivery systems *(see above sections)*.

4.7.14   Analytical techniques

Analytical techniques are essential for qualitative and quantitative analysis of drug substances, excipients, and impurities in dosage forms. Techniques used are UV, FTIR, Mass, NMR, titration, chromatography techniques, etc (see above section).

4.7.15   Microbiological study

To ensure the safety and effectiveness of the product, microbiological evaluation of semisolid/solid dosage forms includes determining if microorganisms such as bacteria, fungi, and other pathogens are present. This test guarantees that no dangerous bacteria in the formulation could infect patients or cause negative effects. According to pharmacopeial standards and legal criteria, sterility testing, microbial enumeration, microbiological limit testing, and tests for particular pathogens are carried out. For instance, An ointment is applied topically to heal skin infections. Microbiological analysis verifies that no bacteria or fungi in the ointment could exacerbate the infection or endanger the patient (126).

4.7.16   Stability studies

Stability studies assess dosage forms' physical, chemical, and microbiological stability over time under various environmental conditions, ensuring product quality and shelf life (*see above section*).

4.7.17   Cell line studies

The way that solid dosage forms interact with human or animal cells is evaluated by cell line research. They help in formulation development and safety assessment by offering insight into the toxicity, mechanisms of action, and efficacy of drugs. Methods: Gene expression analysis employing methods including alarmable assay and qPCR, proliferation assays, and cell viability tests (MTT) (127).

4.8   In vitro testing

In vitro studies provide predictive information on dosage form drug release, diffusion, and permeation characteristics, guiding formulation optimization and predicting in vivo performance. In vitro studies commonly utilized excised human or animal skin. While, when biological skin is not available, synthetic membranes can be used

Important role:

- Simulation of skin
- Quality control
- Toxicity screening
- Designing and developing new products (128).

a.   Drug release testing

The phenomenon known as "drug release" refers to the movement of drug solutes from their original location within the polymeric system to the outside of the polymer and ultimately to the release media. The usual objectives have been to (i) predict drug availability in the early stages of product development; (ii) meet batch standards; (iii) assess formulation parameters and dosage form manufacturing techniques; (iv) bolster product label claims; and (v) comply with regulatory requirements and compendial standards. Information regarding the product's in vivo performance is essential. Drug release testing is attractive because it facilitates the assessment of long-term release throughout the R&D process more quickly (129).

b.   Skin permeation/ diffusion study

Their permeability strongly influences the ability of pharmacological compounds to pass across biological membranes. The inability of many drugs to reach the intended site, the requirement for high drug concentrations to produce the desired effect, low bioavailability, and poor absorption limit their effectiveness. Their high drug load, enhanced permeability, and biocompatibility may make them the perfect delivery mechanism when creating gels or ointments. Franz diffusion cells have become a prominent research tool for determining skin permeability, providing valuable information on how the skin, medicine, and formulation interact. Benefits of using Franz Cells, a well-liked method for evaluating drug penetration, include (i) less tissue handling, (ii) no requirement for ongoing sample collection, and (iii) the small quantity of medication required for analysis (130).

c.   Skin retention studies

As crucial as transdermal permeability, the skin retention amount has been accepted as an essential parameter for assessing topical efficacy or skin irritation. It indicates the effect of formulation on in vitro performance. Topical therapies frequently anticipate high levels of skin retention and less penetration into the bloodstream, which is preferred to lower the risk of systemic side effects. Techniques: Franz diffusion cell apparatus is frequently used for assessing in vitro testing (131).

4.9 Practical aspects for conducting an animal study

Preclinical, in-vivo, animal research and animal experimentation are other terms used in animal studies. Research done on live things, or "in vivo" studies, provides valuable insights into the effects of drugs or the course of disease. However, a complex model can more precisely evaluate a drug candidate's safety, toxicity, and efficacy. Furthermore, scientists can now accurately mimic human diseases in animals because of advancements in gene editing. Researchers can understand significant biological and physiological processes using animals in fundamental research. This knowledge could help us avoid, identify, treat, and cure illnesses more effectively. Similar to human clinical studies, animal experiments reveal similar risk factors.

4.9.1 *Significance of animal experimentation in the current era*

- Allows us to study mechanisms involved in diseased states' emergence, progress, and systemic manifestations.
- They have greater clinical relevance.
- Give more specific and detailed results.
- Give insight into the underlying genetics of the diseased state and the hereditary pattern (132).
- Animal models are fundamental in understanding rare diseases' prognosis and treatment.

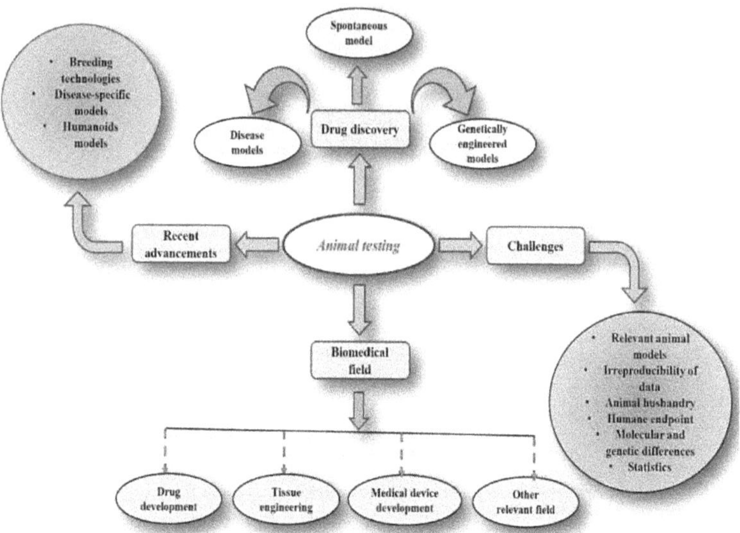

Image 4.6: Animal testing: recent advancements and challenges (Own creation).

i.   Rodent model

Rats and mice are the most common rodent models used in illness research. Deep insight into the study of diabetes, cancer, Alzheimer's disease, wound healing, and other behavioral or neurological disorders has been made possible by the majority of rodent models. Because of their similar illness manifestation to human disease, convenience of availability at cheaper costs, relatively lax animal ethics rules, simplicity of care and handling, shorter reproductive cycle, etc., rodent models are prominent in biomedical research. Furthermore, their reduced lifespan facilitates studies on the inheritance of diseases, developmental biology, and the consequences of genetic engineering. In addition to mice and rats, guinea pigs and hamsters are also frequently utilized as animal models (133). Genetically modified models (GEM) are widely used in biomedical research in addition to wild forms, and they can be obtained according to experimental design. These GEMs are better adapted to researching the fluctuating stages of human illnesses. Numerous organizations, such as the Mutant Mouse Regional Resource Centers and the Rat Resource and Research Center, are leading repositories for conserving and disseminating rodent models. Because of their over 95% genetic resemblance to humans, rodents are extremely important in biological research (134).

ii.   Nonrodent model

Among nonrodent species, rabbits, zebrafish, and fruit flies are most popular in biomedical research. Rabbits are routinely used for atherosclerosis studies, immunology, reproduction, ocular diseases, and osteoporosis (135). It is also widely used to produce polyclonal antibiotics. Zebrafish is extensively used in research related to developmental biology, biochemistry, and molecular biology (136). Due to the presence of orthologous human genes, rapid development, large clutches of egg-laying capacity, and shorter life span, the use of zebrafish as animal models has grown exponentially over the years. Other nonrodent species, like reptiles and amphibians, are frequently used in studies related to evolution and ecology (137).

4.9.2   Ethical guidelines while conducting the animal study

For research involving animal use in biomedical sciences, the 3Rs concept (replacement, reduction, and refinement) needs to be followed (138). The European Directive 2010/63 stipulates that replacement must be the primary goal. Substituting animals with non-animal techniques tends to reduce the use of animals. As long as it appears that using animals is inevitable, the goal is to employ as few animals as possible to provide a meaningful result. Lastly, to optimize the data gathered from animal research, extra attention must be given to improving animal welfare and legitimate applications. Only well-thought-out planning, the animal facility's condition, the specific species' compatibility in the intended experiments, and a skilled team of specialist professionals involved in animal handling, maintenance, and dose administrations should be used to ensure animal studies (139). All animal studies reported for publication must comply with the animal research: reporting of in-vivo experiments (ARRIVE) guidelines (140). The planning research and experimental procedures on animals: recommendations for excellence (PREPARE) guidelines must further be followed before conducting animal studies.

The PREPARE guidelines contain checklists and reminders that should be followed before and during carrying out animal studies (141). The organizations including the Committee for Purpose of Control and Supervision on Animal Experiments, the International Conference on Harmonization of Technical Requirements for Registration of Pharmaceuticals for Human Use (ICH), the National Institute of Health, and the Organization for Economic Cooperation and Development provide guidelines for the animal welfare like animal house maintenance, breeding, feeding, transportation, and mainly for their use in scientific experimentation (142)According to the Institutional Animal Care and Use Committee (IACUC), the protocols are appropriate and adhere to the 3Rs, which represent the standards for humane experimental techniques.

Table 4.12: PREPARE checklist for conducting animal research.

A step-by-step guide for PhD programme

Topic	Recommendation
(A) Formulation of the study	
1. Literature searches	☐ Form a clear hypothesis, with primary and secondary outcomes. ☐ Consider the use of systematic reviews. ☐ Decide upon databases and information specialists to be consulted, and construct search terms. ☐ Assess the relevance of the species to be used, its biology and suitability to answer the experimental questions with the least suffering, and its welfare needs. ☐ Assess the reproducibility and translatability of the project.
2. Legal issues	☐ Consider how the research is affected by relevant legislation for animal research and other areas, e.g. animal transport, occupational health and safety. ☐ Locate relevant guidance documents (e.g. EU guidance on project evaluation).
3. Ethical issues, harm-benefit assessment and humane endpoints	☐ Construct a lay summary. ☐ In dialogue with ethics committees, consider whether statements about this type of research have already been produced. ☐ Address the 3Rs (replacement, reduction, refinement) and the 3Ss (good science, good sense, good sensibilities). ☐ Consider pre-registration and the publication of negative results. ☐ Perform a harm-benefit assessment and justify any likely animal harm. ☐ Discuss the learning objectives, if the animal use is for educational or training purposes. ☐ Allocate a severity classification to the project. ☐ Define objective, easily measurable and unequivocal humane endpoints. ☐ Discuss the justification, if any, for death as an end-point.
4. Experimental design and statistical analysis	☐ Consider pilot studies, statistical power and significance levels. ☐ Define the experimental unit and decide upon animal numbers. ☐ Choose methods of randomisation, prevent observer bias, and decide upon inclusion and exclusion criteria.

4.9.3   Guide to conducting animal research

i.   Define research objectives

It's imperative to specify the goal of any research before starting. This entails stating the precise objectives and queries that the research seeks to answer. These goals act as a road map for research projects, directing them toward significant results.

ii.   Literature review

- Clearly state your hypothesis and its primary and secondary results.

- Take into account applying systematic reviews.

- Choose which databases and information experts to contact, then create search phrases.

- Evaluate the species' use, biology, suitability for addressing the research objectives with the least amount of suffering, and welfare requirements.

- Evaluate the project's repeatability and translateability. (141).

iii.   Design the protocol

Developing a detailed research protocol is essential for ensuring the consistency and reproducibility of the study. This includes outlining the animal model, experimental procedures, sample size determination, data collection methods, and statistical analysis plan. A well-designed protocol provides a structured framework for conducting the research and minimizes potential biases (143).

iv.   Ethics committee approval

Researching animals requires approval from an ethics commission (EC). The study protocol must be submitted for review to ensure compliance with ethical standards and animal welfare recommendations (https://www.pristynresearch.com/services/details/9/ec-registration-services).

Getting ethical permission shows that one is dedicated to ethically doing research and protecting the welfare of study animals. For instance, your research proposal must be submitted for evaluation to the Institutional Animal Care and Use Committee (IACUC) or a comparable regulatory authority (144).

v.   Animal procurement

Selecting the appropriate animal model is critical in designing an animal study. This involves considering factors such as physiological similarity to humans, availability, ethical considerations, and relevance to the research objectives (145). All animals must be acquired lawfully as per the CPCSEA guidelines. Procure animals from reputable suppliers or breeding facilities. Consider factors such as species, age, sex, and health status to ensure consistency and reliability in your study. Choose an animal model based on your research purpose, such as:

a.   **Cancer**
- Mouse xenograft models
- Transgenic mouse models
- Chemically induced carcinogenesis models

b.   **Diabetes**
- Streptozotocin-induced diabetic rat model
- Genetically modified mouse models
- Spontaneous diabetic models

c.   **Acne**
- Porcine sebaceous gland model

- Rabbit ear model
- Murine models

d. **Cardiovascular Disease**: Apolipoprotein E-deficient (ApoE-/) mice

e. **Neurological Disorders**: Transgenic mouse models

f. **Inflammatory disease**

- Complete Freund's adjuvant (CFA) induced inflammation
- Dextran sodium sulfate (DSS)-induced colitis
- Carrageenan-induced paw oedema
- Rat models
- Rabbit models
- Air pouch model.

vi. Animal care and housing

Proper housing and care are necessary to ensure the welfare of research animals for the duration of the study. This entails preserving ideal living circumstances, including proper nutrition, temperature, humidity, cleanliness, and veterinary care. According to CPCSEA standards,

- Animals should be fed with palatable, non-contaminated, and nutritionally adequate food with fresh, potable water daily.
- Food should be provided in sufficient amounts to ensure normal growth in immature animals and to maintain normal body weight, reproduction, and lactation in adults.
- Adequate ventilation and a comfortable environment should be provided. Air conditioning is an effective means of regulating these environmental parameters.

- Temperature and humidity control prevents variations due to changing climatic conditions. Considering the variations in the number of room occupants, the range should always be within or approximately between 18 and 29°C (64.4 to 84.2 °F).

- It is recommended that the relative humidity be maintained between 30% and 70%.

- Fluorescent lights are an efficient lighting option, with less than 400 lux being ideal for rodent facilities.

- Animal attendants must be appropriately trained and skilled in their assigned tasks. Animal houses must be in a calm area free from traffic noise, the grounds must be maintained clean and hygienic, and the animals must be sheltered from drought and extreme weather.

- A veterinarian or someone with expertise or experience in laboratory animal sciences and medicine is responsible for providing adequate veterinary care. (146,147).

vii.   Experimental procedures

It is essential to conduct experimental procedures according to the approved protocol. Proper anesthesia, analgesia, and humane handling techniques minimize pain, distress, and discomfort. Procedures must be standardized to maintain consistency and reliability across experiments.

viii.   Data collection and analysis

Systematic data collection and analysis are necessary for the research to yield relevant conclusions. This entails documenting measurements, observations, and experimental results in line with the established protocol. After that, statistical analysis techniques are used to evaluate the data and come to reliable results (148).

ix.   Monitoring and care

Regularly monitor animals for signs of distress, illness, or adverse effects related to the experiment. Provide veterinary care as needed and implement humane endpoints to minimize suffering.

x.   Reporting and publication

Prepare research findings for publication in peer-reviewed journals, adhering to ethical standards and reporting guidelines. Share data and methodologies to promote transparency and reproducibility in scientific research.

4.9.4   *Safety Measures During Animal Study*

Several precautions should be taken to ensure the welfare of research animals and the validity of research outcomes. These include:

a.   **Ethical compliance**:

- Adhere strictly to CPCSEA guidelines and obtain requisite approvals from institutional animal ethics committees before commencing any animal study.

- Ensure that research protocols are designed to minimize pain, distress, and suffering in animals, aligning with the principles of the 3Rs.

b.   **Personnel training and accreditation**:

- Provide comprehensive training to all personnel involved in animal experimentation, covering ethical considerations, proper handling techniques, and safety protocols.

c.   **Animal welfare standards**:

- Maintain animal housing facilities, ensuring appropriate temperature, humidity, ventilation, and lighting conditions.

- Provide clean and comfortable housing, adequate space, and environmental enrichment to promote animals' physical and psychological well-being.
- Because perishable foods, such meats, fruits, and vegetables, can cause chemical and microbial contamination and alter the amount of nutrients ingested, care should be taken when feeding them.
- Diet should be free from heavy metals (e.g., lead, arsenic, cadmium, nickel, mercury), naturally occurring toxins, and other contaminants.

d. **Health monitoring and veterinary care**:

- Implement regular health monitoring programs to promptly detect and address any signs of animal illness or distress.
- Provide access to veterinary care and ensure that qualified veterinarians are available for consultation and treatment as needed.

e. **Biosecurity measures**:

- Implement stringent biosecurity protocols to prevent the introduction and spread of infectious diseases within animal facilities.
- Control access to animal housing areas, establish quarantine procedures for newly arrived animals, and maintain strict hygiene practices.

f. **Anaesthesia and analgesia**:

- Use proper sedation, analgesia, and anesthetic treatments to reduce discomfort and suffering during experimental procedures.

- Ascertain that anesthesia methods are applied by qualified professionals and customized to meet the requirements of each species and individual animal.

g. **Record-keeping and reporting**:

- Maintain accurate and detailed records of all experimental procedures on animals, including anesthesia, surgery, and euthanasia.

- Report any adverse events, unexpected outcomes, or deviations from the approved protocol to the institutional animal ethics committee and CPCSEA authorities promptly (147,149).

4.10 Key considerations for managing clinical trials within institutions

4.10.1 Overview of clinical trials

Research organizations and firms must conduct in-depth preclinical investigations (laboratory and animal studies) to gather information on toxicity and activity before starting clinical trials. Following regulatory authorities' evaluation, human volunteers may be used for safety and toxicity research under close clinical supervision. It is necessary to carry out a lot of clinical investigations with a growing number of participants (150). A subfield of healthcare science and research known as "clinical research" is described as using human subjects to evaluate the efficacy and safety of a medication, biologic (like a vaccination), device (like a vagus nerve stimulator), treatment, or behavioral intervention (151). Finding the safety and efficacy of novel medicines and raising patient outcomes and healthcare standards are the main objectives of clinical trials. There are four stages to the trial:

a. **Phase 1: Safety and dosage**

- Objective: Assess safety and determine optimal dosage.
- Participants: Few healthy volunteers or individuals (20-100).

b. **Phase 2: Efficacy and safety**

- Objective: Further evaluate safety and preliminary efficacy.
- Participants: Larger sample of patients (100-300).

c. **Phase 3: Confirmation and comparative effectiveness**

- Objective: Confirm efficacy and safety and compare with standard treatment or placebo.
- Participants: Hundreds to thousands of patients (300-3,000).

d. **Phase 4: Post-Marketing Surveillance**

- Objective: Monitor long-term safety and effectiveness in real-world settings.
- Participants: A large population prescribed the approved product (thousands) (152).

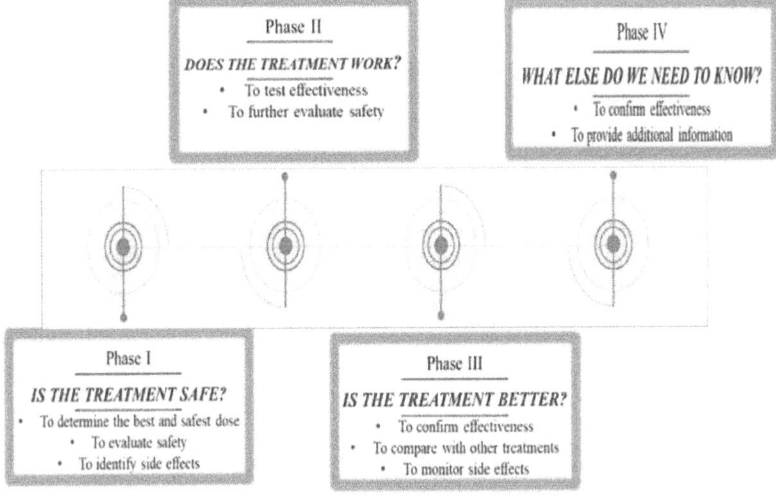

Image 4.7: Phases of clinical trials.

Different types of clinical trials, such as observational, adaptive, and randomised controlled trials, are available to address distinct research problems and aims. Their importance comes from offering data based on evidence to support regulatory approvals, directing clinical practice, and expanding our understanding of medicine (153).

4.10.2   Planning and conducting of clinical trials

a)   Systematic literature reviews

Clearly defining the investigation's study objectives is vital while conducting clinical trials. The goal should be crystal clear in terms of our course of action. We can then proceed with a review of the literature. The authors of published papers will be notified about the current clinical data on a study issue through systematic literature reviews. This is crucial in minimizing ineffective attempts and assessing the intended research. A literature review is essential in starting a new research project. Researchers can learn numerous things from a meticulously carried out and carefully evaluated systematic review that incorporates in-process experiments (154).

b)   Setting up protocol

A protocol outlines the study's objectives, design, methodology, and procedures in detail. Critical components of a protocol include:

- Background and rationale
- Study objectives
- Study design
- Methods
- Statistical considerations
- Ethical considerations
- References.

c)   *Ethics committee approval*

A clinical research project involving human subjects must first have approval from an institutional review board (IRB) or an EC. The EC wants to ensure the study complies with moral guidelines, upholds participant rights, and reduces risks. Researchers usually submit a comprehensive study protocol, which the EC reviews for compliance with regulations, ethical issues, and scientific validity. The EC approves the trial once it concludes that it satisfies its requirements. Approval is required before beginning any research involving human subjects.

d)   *Patient recruitment and informed consent*

Patient recruitment involves identifying and enrolling eligible participants in the study. Recruitment strategies may vary depending on the study's target population, inclusion criteria, and available resources.

Standard recruitment methods include:

- Referral from healthcare providers.
- Advertisement through flyers, posters, or online platforms.
- Direct contact with potential participants through clinics or community outreach.

Recruitment efforts should adhere to ethical principles, such as avoiding coercion or undue influence and providing accurate information about the study (155). Apart from that, researchers must obtain informed consent from each participant or their legally authorized representative before enrolment, which provides participants with detailed information about the study, including its objectives, procedures, risks, benefits, and alternatives.

e)   *Study design*

It includes the following steps:

Selection of site: The correct location for clinical trials ensures a smooth and efficient study implementation. Several things need to be considered to ensure that the required facilities—whether hospitals or institutions—are available. The study's infrastructure, including patient care facilities, laboratory services, and data collecting and analysis equipment, should support the location of choice. Experienced personnel who can accurately and morally administer the trial protocols must work at the site. It's also critical to assess participant accessibility and adherence to legal requirements. Through careful site selection, researchers can increase the chances of a fruitful and significant clinical trial (156).

Registration of clinical trial on the CTRI website: Registration on the Clinical Trials Registry of India (CTRI) (https://ctri.nic.in/Clinicaltrials/login.php) typically occurs after enrolling the first subjects into the study. Registration is a must, no matter its size. It's like an extensive database for all trial results, keeping things transparent. This registration is legal, ensuring everyone knows about ongoing and finished trials. People need this info to understand how research is going. Patient details are kept private, and nothing personal gets out. This whole process keeps things in line with rules and builds trust in research integrity, showing trials are on track (157).

Sample size: When a study is planned, the sample size must be estimated; a sample that is too big is unnecessary and unethical, while a sample that is too small is unscientific and unethical. Using statistical software, the necessary sample size can be calculated based on certain assumptions (158). It is like a puzzle where all these pieces must fit together for reliable results.

Inclusion and exclusion criteria: In clinical trials, eligibility criteria are a crucial section as they define the patient population included in the study. These criteria were often customized to evaluate a treatment's effectiveness in a well-defined population. An essential feature of the target audience that the investigators will utilize to address their research question is identified as inclusion criteria. The characteristics of potential study participants who match the inclusion criteria nonetheless have extra traits that might hamper the study's success or increase their risk of adverse consequences, which are known as exclusion criteria.

Grouping of Subjects and Randomization: For reliable findings, group subjects in clinical studies are based on variables such as age, gender, weight, etc. This makes it possible to accurately assess the treatment's effects across a range of demographic groups. It's also important to randomize; this entails putting individuals in groups at random rather than by choice. This indicates that the outcomes accurately reflect the treatment's effectiveness and help to eliminate bias. Thus, by carefully assigning people to groups and generating random assignments, researchers can obtain trustworthy information on how well the treatment is working (159).

Study procedure: The study procedure should be followed according to protocol while conducted with the adherence to ethical guidelines such as ICMR National ethical guidelines for biomedical and health research involving human participants, ICH GCP Guidelines, new drugs & clinical trials rules 2019, declaration of Helsinki and by other applicable guidelines. Clinical trials encompass crucial procedures such as evaluating the participants' health status, conducting laboratory assessments, administering the investigational product (IP), and analyzing plasma samples. These steps are pivotal in ensuring thorough evaluation, accurate data collection, and adherence to the trial protocol (160).

Data management and monitoring*:* Data management and monitoring involve the systematic collection, storage, and analysis of study data to ensure accuracy, reliability, and compliance with regulatory standards. This process includes establishing data collection tools, such as case report forms (CRFs), electronic data capture (EDC) systems, or other data management platforms. Additionally, data monitoring involves ongoing review and verification of collected data to identify discrepancies, errors, or protocol deviations (161).

Safety and ADR management: To quickly record and assess any adverse events or ADRs that arise during the trial, safety monitoring procedures, such as adverse event reporting systems, must be implemented. Furthermore, for the sake of participant safety and regulatory compliance, safety data is routinely reviewed by a clinical events committee (CEC) or independent data safety monitoring board (DSMB) (162).

Data analysis: Data analysis involves transforming raw data into meaningful insights, identifying patterns, trends, and relationships, and drawing conclusions based on statistical or qualitative methods. Statistical analysis is commonly used to quantify relationships between variables, assess the significance of findings, and test hypotheses. Qualitative techniques, such as content or thematic analysis, are employed to interpret textual or narrative data, providing in-depth understanding and contextual insights. Data analysis often involves the use of specialized software tools, such as statistical packages (e.g., SPSS,

SAS, R) or qualitative analysis software (e.g., NVivo, Atlas. ti), to facilitate efficient and accurate analysis (163).

Dissemination and publication: Develop plans for disseminating trial results through peer-reviewed publications, presentations at scientific conferences, and other relevant forums. Ensure transparency and accountability in reporting trial findings, including publication of results regardless of outcome. Also, the trial results are submitted to the CTRI website for transparency and accessibility to the public (164).

4.11 References

1.   Chaudhari Rahul B. A Review On Research Methodology – I. 2023.

2. CR Kothari. Research technology methods and techniques. In: 2nd ed. New Age International (P) Ltd. New Delhi;

3. Marczyk GR, DeMatteo D, Festinger D. Essentials of research design and methodology. John Wiley & Sons; 2010.

4. Awaisu A, Mukhalalati B, Ibrahim MIM. Research Designs and Methodologies Related to Pharmacy Practice.

5. Tripodi, Stephen, Kimberly Bender. Descriptive studies. In: The handbook of social work research methods. 2010. p. 120–30.

6. Seixas BV, Smith N, Mitton C. The Qualitative Descriptive Approach in International Comparative Studies: Using Online Qualitative Surveys. Int J Health Policy Manag. 2017 Dec 23;7(9):778–81.

7. Lim EP, Chen H, Chen G. Business Intelligence and Analytics: Research Directions. ACM Trans Manage Inf Syst. 2013 Jan;3(4):1–10.

8. Poling A, Methot LL, LeSage MG. Fundamentals of behavior analytic research. In Springer Science & Business Media; 1995.

9. Mahmoud Rababah. What is applied research? 2023;

10. Hedrick, Terry E.., Bickman, Leonard., Rog, Debra J. Applied Research Design: A Practical Guide. In United States: SAGE Publications; 1993.

11. Tolley EE, Ulin PR, Mack N, Robinson ET, Succop SM. Qualitative Methods in Public Health: A Field Guide for Applied Research. In John Wiley & Sons; 2016.

12. Corey SM. Action Research, Fundamental Research, and Educational Practices. Teachers College Record. 1949 May;50(8):1–4.

13. Disman, D., Ali, M. & Syaom Barliana, M. The Use of Quantitative Research Method and Statistical Data Analysis In Dissertation: An Evaluation Study. International Journal of Education. 2017;10(1):46–52.

14. Creswell JW, Poth CN. Qualitative inquiry and research design: Choosing among five approaches. In SAGE Publications; 2016.

15. Ahmed V, Opoku A, Aziz Z, editors. Research methodology in the built environment: a selection of case studies. Abingdon, Oxon: Routledge; 2016.

16. Tobi H, Kampen JK. Research design: the methodology for interdisciplinary research framework. Qual Quant. 2018 May;52(3):1209–25.

17. Mora M, Gelman O, Paradice D, Cervantes F. The Case for Conceptual Research in Information Systems.

18. Ranjan Kumar. Experimental Method: Advantages and limitations.

19. Verma, G. and Mishra, M.K. Pharmaceutical pre-formulation studies in formulation and development of new dosage form: A review. Int J Pharma Res Rev. 2016;5(10).

20. Ahirwar K, Shukla R. Preformulation Studies: A Versatile Tool in Formulation Design. In: Shukla R, Kuznetsov A, Ali A, editors. Drug Formulation Design [Internet]. IntechOpen; 2023 [cited 2024 Mar 28]. Available from: https://www.intechopen.com/chapters/86211

21. Kulkarni, S., Sharma, S.B. and Agrawal, A. Preformulation-A Foundation For Formulation Development. International Journal of Pharmaceutical, Chemical & Biological Sciences. 2015;5(2).

22. Chaurasia, G. A review of pharmaceutical preformulation studies in formulation and development of new drug molecules. IJPSR. 2016;7(6):2313–20.

23. Belz S. [The pharmacopoeia. An important pillar of drug safety]. Bundesgesundheitsblatt Gesundheitsforschung Gesundheitsschutz. 2006 Dec;49(12):1205–11.

24. Kirtawade R, Salve P, Seervi C, Kulkarni A, Dhabale P. Simultaneous UV spectrophotometric method for estimation of paracetamol and nimesulide in tablet dosage form. International Journal of ChemTech Research. 2010;2(2):818-821.

25. Khan A, Naquvi KJ, Haider MF, Khan MA. Quality by design- a newer technique for pharmaceutical product development. Intelligent Pharmacy. 2024 Feb;2(1):122–9.

26. Chavda H, Patel C, Anand I. Biopharmaceutics classification system. Syst Rev Pharm. 2010;1(1):62.

27. Garg S, Kandarapu R, Vermani K, Tambwekar KR, Garg A, Waller DP, et al. Development Pharmaceutics of Microbicide Formulations. Part I: Preformulation Considerations and Challenges. AIDS Patient Care and STDs. 2003 Jan;17(1):17–32.

28. Teekamp, N. Protein delivery from polymeric matrices: From pre-formulation stabilization studies to site-specific delivery. 2018.

29. Feroz Jameel. Development of Biopharmaceutical Drug-Device Products. Germany: Springer International Publishing. 2020;

30. Dooley, N., Ford, S. J., Prasad, E., Elliott, M., & Halbert, G (last). Abstracts from the UK-Pharmsci Conference, 1–3 September 2010. Journal of Pharmacy and Pharmacology. 2010 Sep 3;62(10):1201–516.

31. Clapham D. Chapter 11. Presentational and Organoleptic Aspects of Formulation. In: Tovey GD, editor. Drug Development and

Pharmaceutical Science [Internet]. Cambridge: Royal Society of Chemistry; 2022 [cited 2024 Mar 28]. p. 287–320. Available from: http://ebook.rsc.org/?DOI=10.1039/9781839165603-00287

32. Gopinath R, Naidu RAS. Pharmaceutical Preformulation Studies – Current Review. 2010;2.

33. Lian B, Yalkowsky SH. Molecular Geometry and Melting Point Related Properties. Ind Eng Chem Res. 2012 Dec 26;51(51):16750–4.

34. Saal C, Petereit AC. Optimizing solubility: Kinetic versus thermodynamic solubility temptations and risks. European Journal of Pharmaceutical Sciences. 2012 Oct;47(3):589–95.

35. Behnood A, Van Tittelboom K, De Belie N. Methods for measuring pH in concrete: A review. Construction and Building Materials. 2016 Feb;105:176–88.

36. Daina A, Michielin O, Zoete V. iLOGP: A Simple, Robust, and Efficient Description of n -Octanol/Water Partition Coefficient for Drug Design Using the GB/SA Approach. J Chem Inf Model. 2014 Dec 22;54(12):3284–301.

37. Brog JP, Chanez CL, Crochet A, Fromm KM. Polymorphism, what it is and how to identify it: a systematic review. RSC Adv. 2013;3(38):16905.

38. Newman AW, Reutzel-Edens SM, Zografi G. Characterization of active pharmaceutical ingredients "hygroscopic" properties. Journal of Pharmaceutical Sciences. 2008 Mar;97(3):1047–59.

39. Xie H, Gong G, Wu Y, Liu Y, Wang Y. Research on the Hygroscopicity of a Composite Hygroscopic Material and its Influence on Indoor Thermal and Humidity Environment. Applied Sciences. 2018 Mar 13;8(3):430.

40. Cabiscol R, Shi H, Wünsch I, Magnanimo V, Finke JH, Luding S, et al. Effect of particle size on powder compaction and tablet strength using limestone. Advanced Powder Technology. 2020 Mar;31(3):1280–9.

41. Harahap U, Marianne M, Yuandani Y, Laila L. Preformulation Study of Pugun Tano (Curanga fel-terrae [Lour.] Merr) Ethanolic Extract Granule Mass in Capsule as Hepatoprotective Drug. Open Access Maced J Med Sci. 2019 Nov 14;7(22):3729–32.

42. Akseli I, Hilden J, Katz JM, Kelly RC, Kramer TT, Mao C, et al. Reproducibility of the Measurement of Bulk/Tapped Density of Pharmaceutical Powders Between Pharmaceutical Laboratories. Journal of Pharmaceutical Sciences. 2019 Mar;108(3):1081–4.

43. Hill J, Sleep B, Drake J, Fryer M. The Effect of Intraparticle Porosity and Interparticle Voids on the Hydraulic Properties of Soilless Media. Vadose Zone Journal. 2019 Jan;18(1):1–13.

44. Moravkar KK, Korde SD, Bhairav BA, Shinde SB, Kakulade SV, Chalikwar SS. Traditional and Advanced Flow Characterization Techniques: A Platform Review for Development of Solid Dosage Form. ijps [Internet]. 2020 [cited 2024 Mar 28];82(6). Available from: https://www.ijpsonline.com/articles/traditional-and-advanced-flow-characterization-techniques-a-platform-review-for-development-of-solid-dosage-form-4047.html

45. Baranov MV, Kumar M, Sacanna S, Thutupalli S, Van Den Bogaart G. Modulation of Immune Responses by Particle Size and Shape. Front Immunol. 2021 Feb 12;11:607945.

46. Finlay WH, Darquenne C. Particle Size Distributions. Journal of Aerosol Medicine and Pulmonary Drug Delivery. 2020 Aug 1;33(4):178–80.

47. Akhtar K, Khan SA, Khan SB, Asiri AM. Scanning Electron Microscopy: Principle and Applications in Nanomaterials Characterization. In: Sharma SK, editor. Handbook of Materials Characterization [Internet]. Cham: Springer International Publishing; 2018 [cited 2024 Mar 28]. p. 113–45. Available from: http://link.springer.com/10.1007/978-3-319-92955-2_4

48. Asadi Asadabad M, Jafari Eskandari M. Transmission Electron Microscopy as Best Technique for Characterization in Nanotechnology. Synthesis and Reactivity in Inorganic, Metal-Organic, and Nano-Metal Chemistry. 2015 Mar 4;45(3):323–6.

49. Kumar A, Singh P, Nanda A. Hot stage microscopy and its applications in pharmaceutical characterization. Appl Microsc. 2020 Dec;50(1):12.

50. Bittelli M, Pellegrini S, Olmi R, Andrenelli MC, Simonetti G, Borrelli E, et al. Experimental evidence of laser diffraction accuracy for particle size analysis. Geoderma. 2022 Mar;409:115627.

51. Farkas N, Kramar JA. Dynamic light scattering distributions by any means. J Nanopart Res. 2021 May;23(5):120.

52. Chaloupkova, Veronika, Tatiana Ivanova, and Bohumil Havrland (last). Sieve analysis of biomass: an accurate method for determination of particle size distribution. 2016;25–7.

53. Zhang W, Hu Y, Choi G, Liang S, Liu M, Guan W. Microfluidic multiple cross-correlated Coulter counter for improved particle size analysis. Sensors and Actuators B: Chemical. 2019 Oct; 296:126615.

54. Yokojima S, Takashima R, Asada H, Miyahara T. Impacts of particle shape on sedimentation of particles. European Journal of Mechanics - B/Fluids. 2021 Sep; 89:323–31.

55. Brame, Jonathon A., and Christopher S. Griggs. Surface area analysis using the Brunauer-Emmett-Teller (BET) method: scientific operation procedure series: SOP-C. 2016;

56. Palacios, M., Kazemi-Kamyab, H., Mantellato, S. and Bowen, P. Laser diffraction and gas adsorption techniques. In: A Practical Guide to Microstructural Analysis of Cementitious Materials. 1st ed. CRC Press; 2016. p. 445–83.

57. Epp J. X-ray diffraction (XRD) techniques for materials characterization. In: Materials Characterization Using Nondestructive Evaluation (NDE) Methods [Internet]. Elsevier; 2016 [cited 2024 Mar 28]. p. 81–124. Available from: https://linkinghub.elsevier.com/retrieve/pii/B97800810004030000 43

58. Abd-Elghany M, Klapötke TM. A review of differential scanning calorimetry technique and its importance in the field of energetic materials. Physical Sciences Reviews. 2018 Apr 25;3(4):20170103.

59. Ferreira AP, Gamble JF, Leane MM, Park H, Olusanmi D, Tobyn M. Enhanced Understanding of Pharmaceutical Materials Through Advanced Characterisation and Analysis. AAPS PharmSciTech. 2018 Nov;19(8):3462–80.

60. Schinke C, Christian Peest P, Schmidt J, Brendel R, Bothe K, Vogt MR, et al. Uncertainty analysis for the coefficient of band-to-band absorption of crystalline silicon. AIP Advances. 2015 Jun 1;5(6):067168.

61. Yuan L, Gu H, Zeng J, Pillutla RC, Ji QC. Application of in-sample calibration curve methodology for regulated bioanalysis: Critical considerations in method development, validation, and sample analysis. Journal of Pharmaceutical and Biomedical Analysis. 2020 Jan; 177:112844.

62. Mohamed MA, Jaafar J, Ismail AF, Othman MHD, Rahman MA. Fourier Transform Infrared (FTIR) Spectroscopy. In: Membrane Characterization [Internet]. Elsevier; 2017 [cited 2024 Mar 29]. p. 3–29. Available from: https://linkinghub.elsevier.com/retrieve/pii/B97804446377650000 12

63. Durowoju IB, Bhandal KS, Hu J, Carpick B, Kirkitadze M. Differential Scanning Calorimetry — A Method for

Assessing Protein Antigen's Thermal Stability and Conformation. JoVE. 2017 Mar 4;(121):55262.

64. Leyva-Porras C, Cruz-Alcantar P, Espinosa-Solís V, Martínez-Guerra E, Piñón-Balderrama CI, Compean Martínez I, et al. Application of Differential Scanning Calorimetry (DSC) and Modulated Differential Scanning Calorimetry (MDSC) in Food and Drug Industries. Polymers. 2019 Dec 18;12(1):5.

65. Chadha R, Bhandari S. Drug–excipient compatibility screening—Role of thermoanalytical and spectroscopic techniques. Journal of Pharmaceutical and Biomedical Analysis. 2014 Jan;87:82–97.

66. Wyttenbach N, Birringer C, Alsenz J, Kuentz M. Drug-Excipient Compatibility Testing Using a High-Throughput Approach and Statistical Design. Pharmaceutical Development and Technology. 2005 Jan;10(4):499–505.

67. Gonzalez-Gonzalez M, Yerena-Prieto BJ, Carrera C, Vázquez-Espinosa M, González-de-Peredo AV, García-Alvarado MÁ, et al. Optimization of an Ultrasound-Assisted Extraction Method for the Extraction of Gingerols and Shogaols from Ginger (Zingiber officinale). Agronomy. 2023 Jul 2;13(7):1787.

68. Aashigari S, Goud R, Sneha S, Vykuntam U, Potnuri NR (last). Stability studies of pharmaceutical products.

69. Narayan S, Manupriya C. 10. A- Review- On- Stability- Studies- Of- Pharmaceutical- Products.

70. ICH Q2A: Text on Validation of Analytical Procedures. In: International Conference on Harmonization. Geneva; 1995.

71. Annex 10 Stability testing of active pharmaceutical ingredients and finished pharmaceutical products. ICH. Available from: http://www.ich.org/fileadmin/Public_Web_Site/ICH_Products/Gui delines/Quality/Q1F/Q1F_Explanatory_ Note.pdf

72. Pharmacognostical Studies. Prog Drug Res. 2016;71(5–10).

73. Badal S, Clement YN. Background to pharmacognosy. In: Pharmacognosy [Internet]. Elsevier; 2024 [cited 2024 Apr 2]. p. 3–10. Available from: https://linkinghub.elsevier.com/retrieve/pii/B97804431865780003 47

74. Balekundri A, Mannur V. Quality control of the traditional herbs and herbal products: a review. Futur J Pharm Sci. 2020 Dec;6(1):67.

75. Yadav M, Chatterji S, Gupta SK, Watal G. Preliminary Phytochemical Screening Of Six Medicinal Plants Used In Traditional Medicine. 6(5).

76. Patil RN. Phytochemical Study and Pharmacological Effects of Dolichandrone falcata Seem. 2021;4(1).
77. Shaikh JR, Patil M. Qualitative tests for preliminary phytochemical screening: An overview. Int J Chem Stud. 2020 Mar 1;8(2):603–8.
78. Wahid S, Tasleem S, Jahangir S. Phytochemical Profiling Of Ethanolic Flower Extract Of Hibiscus Rosa-Sinensis And Evaluation Of Its Antioxidant Potential. World Journal of Pharmaceutical Research. 8(6).
79. Hossain MA, AL-Raqmi KAS, AL-Mijizy ZH, Weli AM, Al-Riyami Q. Study of total phenol, flavonoids contents and phytochemical screening of various leaves crude extracts of locally grown Thymus vulgaris. Asian Pacific Journal of Tropical Biomedicine. 2013 Sep;3(9):705–10.
80. Moulishankar, Anguraj, Prasanna Ganesan, Madhivanan Elumalai, and Karthikeyan Lakshmanan. Significance of TLC and HPTLC in phytochemical screening of herbal drugs. J Glob Pharma Technol. 2020; 12:30–45.
81. Koparde AA. Phyto Active Compounds From Herbal Plant Extracts: Its Extraction, Isolation And Characterization. WJPR. 2017 Aug 1;1186–205.
82. Kumar A, Gupta GD, Raikwar S. Artificial Intelligence Technologies used for the Assessment of PharmaceuticalExcipients. CPD. 2024 Feb;30(6):407–9.
83. Tyagi S, Pathak A, Sharma V, Katyal G, Bhardwaj A, Sharma L, et al. AI-assisted Formulation Design for Improved Drug Delivery and Bioavailability.
84. Wang N, Sun H, Dong J, Ouyang D. PharmDE: A new expert system for drug-excipient compatibility evaluation. International Journal of Pharmaceutics. 2021 Sep; 607:120962.
85. Paul D, Sanap G, Shenoy S, Kalyane D, Kalia K, Tekade RK. Artificial intelligence in drug discovery and development. Drug Discovery Today. 2021 Jan;26(1):80–93.
86. Ananthu MK, Chintamaneni PK, Shaik SB, Thadipatri R, Mahammed N. Artificial Neural Networks in Optimization of Pharmaceutical Formulations. 2021;
87. Hassanzadeh P, Atyabi F, Dinarvand R. The significance of artificial intelligence in drug delivery system design. Advanced Drug Delivery Reviews. 2019 Nov;151–152:169–90.
88. Madabushi R, Seo P, Zhao L, Tegenge M, Zhu H. Review: Role of Model-Informed Drug Development Approaches in the Lifecycle of

Drug Development and Regulatory Decision-Making. Pharm Res. 2022 Aug;39(8):1669–80.

89. R. Rajesh *. Importance Of Drug Excipient Compatibility Studies By Using Or Utilizing Or Employing Various Analytical Techniques – An Overview. IJPSR. 13(9).

90. Bokser, A.D. and O'Donnell, P.B. Stability of Pharmaceutical Products. 2013;37.

91. Dave VS, Haware RV, Sangave NA, Sayles M, Popielarczyk M. Drug-Excipient Compatibility Studies in Formulation Development: Current Trends and Techniques.

92. Gala U, Chauhan H. Principles and applications of Raman spectroscopy in pharmaceutical drug discovery and development. Expert Opinion on Drug Discovery. 2015 Feb;10(2):187–206.

93. Muley S, Nandgude T, Poddar S. Extrusion–spheronization a promising pelletization technique: In-depth review. Asian Journal of Pharmaceutical Sciences. 2016 Dec;11(6):684–99.

94. Kharwade R, Badole P, Mahajan N, More S. Toxicity and Surface Modification of Dendrimers: A Critical Review. CDD. 2022 May;19(4):451–65.

95. Kuchekar S, Bhise K. Formulation and development of antipsoriatic herbal gelcream. 2012;71.

96. Salama R, Choi HJ, Almazi J, Traini D, Young P. Generic dry powder inhalers bioequivalence: Batch–to-batch variability insights. Drug Discovery Today. 2022 Nov;27(11):103350.

97. Mr.Siddhant Shelke, Mr. Santosh Waghmare, Dr.Hemant Kamble. A Review on Optimization Techniques in Pharmaceutical Formulation. IJCRT. 2021;9(11): b883–8.

98. Beg S, Swain S, Rahman M, Hasnain MS, Imam SS. Application of Design of Experiments (DoE) in Pharmaceutical Product and Process Optimization. In: Pharmaceutical Quality by Design [Internet]. Elsevier; 2019 [cited 2024 Apr 2]. p. 43–64. Available from: https://linkinghub.elsevier.com/retrieve/pii/B9780128157992000034

99. Sopyan I, Gozali D, Sriwidodo, Guntina RK. Design-Expert Software (Doe): An Application Tool For Optimization In Pharmaceutical Preparations Formulation. Int J App Pharm. 2022 Jul 7;55–63.

100. Taylor CJ, Baker A, Chapman MR, Reynolds WR, Jolley KE, Clemens G, et al. Flow chemistry for process optimisation using design of experiments. J Flow Chem. 2021 Mar;11(1):75–86.

101. Muller PY, Milton MN. The determination and interpretation of the therapeutic index in drug development. Nat Rev Drug Discov. 2012 Oct;11(10):751–61.

102. Mak KK, Wong YH, Pichika MR. Artificial Intelligence in Drug Discovery and Development. In: Hock FJ, Pugsley MK, editors. Drug Discovery and Evaluation: Safety and Pharmacokinetic Assays [Internet]. Cham: Springer International Publishing; 2023 [cited 2024 Apr 2]. p. 1–38. Available from: https://link.springer.com/10.1007/978-3-030-73317-9_92-1

103. Thompson P. Literature Reviews in Applied PhD Theses: Evidence and Problems. In: Hyland K, Diani G, editors. Academic Evaluation [Internet]. London: Palgrave Macmillan UK; 2009 [cited 2024 Mar 21]. p. 50–67. Available from: http://link.springer.com/10.1057/9780230244290_4

104. Kim J, Kim DG, Ryu KH. Enhancing Response Surface Methodology through Coefficient Clipping Based on Prior Knowledge. Processes. 2023 Dec 8;11(12):3392.

105. Bezerra MA, Santelli RE, Oliveira EP, Villar LS, Escaleira LA. Response surface methodology (RSM) as a tool for optimization in analytical chemistry. Talanta. 2008 Sep 15;76(5):965–77.

106. Pereira LMS, Milan TM, Tapia-Blácido DR. Using Response Surface Methodology (RSM) to optimize 2G bioethanol production: A review. Biomass and Bioenergy. 2021 Aug; 151:106166.

107. Mahapatra APK, Saraswat R, Botre M, Paul B, Prasad N. Application of response surface methodology (RSM) in statistical optimization and pharmaceutical characterization of a patient compliance effervescent tablet formulation of an antiepileptic drug levetiracetam. Futur J Pharm Sci. 2020 Dec;6(1):82.

108. Müller ALH, De Oliveira JA, Prestes OD, Adaime MB, Zanella R. Design of experiments and method development. In: Solid-Phase Extraction [Internet]. Elsevier; 2020 [cited 2024 Apr 2]. p. 589–608. Available from: https://linkinghub.elsevier.com/retrieve/pii/B978012816906300024

109. Vera Candioti L, De Zan MM, Cámara MS, Goicoechea HC. Experimental design and multiple response optimization. Using the desirability function in analytical methods development. Talanta. 2014 Jun; 124:123–38.

110. Cano-Lamadrid M, Martínez-Zamora L, Mozafari L, Bueso MC, Kessler M, Artés-Hernández F. Response Surface Methodology to

Optimize the Extraction of Carotenoids from Horticultural By-Products—A Systematic Review. Foods. 2023 Dec 12;12(24):4456.

111. Akhtar M, Zaman M, Siddiqi AZ, Ali H, Khan R, Alvi MN, et al. Response Surface Methodology (RSM) approach to formulate and optimize the bilayer combination tablet of Tamsulosin and Finasteride. Saudi Pharmaceutical Journal. 2024 Mar;32(3):101957.

112. Maqbool A, Mishra MK, Pathak S, Kesharwani A. Semi Solid Dosage Forms Manufacturing: Tools, Critical Process Parameters, Strategies, Optimization, And Recent Advances. 7(11).

113. Adepu S, Ramakrishna S. Controlled Drug Delivery Systems: Current Status and Future Directions. Molecules. 2021 Sep 29;26(19):5905.

114. Himanshu, Sameeksha, Kumar M. A Comprehensive Review on Pharmaceutical Liquid Dosage Form. Act Scie Pharma. 2022 Apr 1;12–24.

115. Mohiuddin A. Extemporaneous Compounding: Selective Pharmacists with Separate Skill. Innov Pharm. 2019 Oct 31;10(4):3.

116. Qwist PK, Sander C, Okkels F, Jessen V, Baldursdottir S, Rantanen J. On-line rheological characterization of semi-solid formulations. European Journal of Pharmaceutical Sciences. 2019 Feb; 128:36–42.

117. Elena O. B, Maria N. A, Michael S. Z, Natalia B. D, Alexander I. B, Ivan I. K. Dermatologic Gels Spreadability Measuring Methods Comparative Study. Int J App Pharm. 2022 Jan 7;164–8.

118. Rompicherla NC, Joshi P, Shetty A, Sudhakar K, Amin HIM, Mishra Y, et al. Design, Formulation, and Evaluation of Aloe vera Gel-Based Capsaicin Transemulgel for Osteoarthritis. Pharmaceutics. 2022 Aug 29;14(9):1812.

119. Li T, Donner AD, Choi CY, Frunzi GP, Morris KR. A statistical support for using spectroscopic methods to validate the content uniformity of solid dosage forms. Journal of Pharmaceutical Sciences. 2003 Jul;92(7):1526–30.

120. Bhoyar PK, Biyani DM, Umekar MJ. Formulation and Characterization of Patient-Friendly Dosage Form of Ondansetron Hydrochloride. Journal of Young Pharmacists. 2010 Jul;2(3):240–6.

121. Karki S, Kim H, Na SJ, Shin D, Jo K, Lee J. Thin films as an emerging platform for drug delivery. Asian Journal of Pharmaceutical Sciences. 2016 Oct;11(5):559–74.

122. Dhakar RC, Maurya SD, Sagar BP, Bhagat S, Prajapati SK, Jain CP. Variables Influencing the Drug Entrapment Efficiency of Microspheres: A Pharmaceutical Review. 2010;

123. Dhadde GS, Mali HS, Raut ID, Nitalikar MM, Bhutkar MA. A Review on Microspheres: Types, Method of Preparation, Characterization and Application. AJPT. 2021 May 13;149–55.

124. Berardi A, Bisharat L, Quodbach J, Abdel Rahim S, Perinelli DR, Cespi M. Advancing the understanding of the tablet disintegration phenomenon – An update on recent studies. International Journal of Pharmaceutics. 2021 Apr; 598:120390.

125. Damian F, Harati M, Schwartzenhauer J, Van Cauwenberghe O, Wettig SD. Challenges of Dissolution Methods Development for Soft Gelatin Capsules. Pharmaceutics. 2021 Feb 4;13(2):214.

126. Jeenathunisa N, Rajan S. In vitro Cytotoxic studies of Saraca asoca bark extracts on HT-29 cancer cell Line. Research Journal of Pharmacy and Technology. 2021;14(1):42–6.

127. Nemes D, Kovács R, Nagy F, Mező M, Poczok N, Ujhelyi Z, et al. Interaction between Different Pharmaceutical Excipients in Liquid Dosage Forms—Assessment of Cytotoxicity and Antimicrobial Activity. Molecules. 2018 Jul 23;23(7):1827.

128. Salamanca C, Barrera-Ocampo A, Lasso J, Camacho N, Yarce C. Franz Diffusion Cell Approach for Pre-Formulation Characterisation of Ketoprofen Semi-Solid Dosage Forms. Pharmaceutics. 2018 Sep 5;10(3):148.

129. Kim Y, Park EJ, Kim TW, Na DH. Recent Progress in Drug Release Testing Methods of Biopolymeric Particulate System. Pharmaceutics. 2021 Aug 23;13(8):1313.

130. Baskar V, I. SM, A. S, S, Ali J, K. ST. Historic Review on Modern Herbal Nanogel Formulation And Delivery Methods. Int J Pharm Pharm Sci. 2018 Oct 1;10(10):1.

131. Tian Q, Quan P, Fang L, Xu H, Liu C. A molecular mechanism investigation of the transdermal/topical absorption classification system on the basis of drug skin permeation and skin retention. International Journal of Pharmaceutics. 2021 Oct; 608:121082.

132. Sakat SS, Bagade O, Mhaske G, Taru P, Sagar M, Rastogi M. Significance of animal experimentation in biomedical research in the current era: Narrative review. J App Pharm Sci [Internet]. 2022 [cited 2024 Apr 3]; Available from: https://japsonline.com/abstract.php?article_id=3696&sts=2

133. Bryda EC. The Mighty Mouse: the impact of rodents on advances in biomedical research. Mo Med. 2013;110(3):207–11.

134. Reza Khorramizadeh M, Saadat F. Animal models for human disease. In: Animal Biotechnology [Internet]. Elsevier; 2020 [cited 2024 Apr 3]. p. 153–71. Available from: https://linkinghub.elsevier.com/retrieve/pii/B97801281171010000 82

135. Rappuoli R. 1885, the first rabies vaccination in humans. Proc Natl Acad Sci USA. 2014 Aug 26;111(34):12273–12273.

136. Peterson RT, Nass R, Boyd WA, Freedman JH, Dong K, Narahashi T. Use of non-mammalian alternative models for neurotoxicological study. NeuroToxicology. 2008 May;29(3):546–55.

137. Hickman DL, Johnson J, Vemulapalli TH, Crisler JR, Shepherd R. Commonly Used Animal Models. In: Principles of Animal Research [Internet]. Elsevier; 2017 [cited 2024 Apr 3]. p. 117–75. Available from: https://linkinghub.elsevier.com/retrieve/pii/B97801280215140000 74

138. Ranganatha N, Kuppast IJ (last). A review on alternatives to animal testing methods in drug development. Int J Pharm Pharm Sci. 2012; 4:28–32.

139. Doke SK, Dhawale SC. Alternatives to animal testing: A review. Saudi Pharmaceutical Journal. 2015 Jul;23(3):223–9.

140. Percie Du Sert N, Ahluwalia A, Alam S, Avey MT, Baker M, Browne WJ, et al. Reporting animal research: Explanation and elaboration for the ARRIVE guidelines 2.0. Boutron I, editor. PLoS Biol. 2020 Jul 14;18(7): e3000411.

141. Smith AJ, Clutton RE, Lilley E, Hansen KEA, Brattelid T. PREPARE: guidelines for planning animal research and testing. Lab Anim. 2018 Apr;52(2):135–41.

142. Rollin BE. Toxicology and New Social Ethics for Animals. Toxicol Pathol. 2003 Jan;31(1_suppl):128–31.

143. Bailoo JD, Reichlin TS, Wurbel H. Refinement of Experimental Design and Conduct in Laboratory Animal Research. ILAR Journal. 2014 Dec 20;55(3):383–91.

144. Portaluppi F, Smolensky MH, Touitou Y. Ethics and Methods for Biological Rhythm Research on Animals And Human Beings. Chronobiology International. 2010 Dec;27(9–10):1911–29.

145. Andersen ML, Winter LMF. Animal models in biological and biomedical research - experimental and ethical concerns. An Acad Bras Ciênc. 2019;91(suppl 1): e20170238.

146. Masedunskas A, Milberg O, Porat-Shliom N, Sramkova M, Wigand T, Amornphimoltham P, et al. Intravital microscopy: A practical

guide on imaging intracellular structures in live animals. BioArchitecture. 2012 Sep;2(5):143–57.

147. Anjani kumar. Committee for the Purpose of Control and Supervision of Experiments on Animals.

148. Vesterinen HM, Sena ES, Egan KJ, Hirst TC, Churolov L, Currie GL, et al. Meta-analysis of data from animal studies: A practical guide. Journal of Neuroscience Methods. 2014 Jan; 221:92–102.

149. Guide for the care and use of laboratory animals. In: Committee for the Update of the Guide for the Care, and Use of Laboratory Animals. National Research Council, Division on Earth, Life Studies, Institute for Laboratory Animal Research; 2010.

150. Wright B. Clinical Trial Phases. In: A Comprehensive and Practical Guide to Clinical Trials [Internet]. Elsevier; 2017 [cited 2024 Apr 4]. p. 11–5. Available from: https://linkinghub.elsevier.com/retrieve/pii/B978012804729300002X

151. Clinical research. 2024; Available from: https://en.wikipedia.org/wiki/Clinical_research

152. Pathan Azher khan. Grab your dream job in pharma:interview questions & answers. 2024.

153. Piantadosi, Steven. Clinical trials: a methodologic perspective. John Wiley & Sons; 2024.

154. Chew BH. Planning and Conducting Clinical Research: The Whole Process. Cureus [Internet]. 2019 Feb 20 [cited 2024 Apr 3]; Available from: https://www.cureus.com/articles/17094-planning-and-conducting-clinical-research-the-whole-process

155. Chaudhari N, Ravi R, Gogtay N, Thatte U. Recruitment and retention of the participants in clinical trials: Challenges and solutions. Perspect Clin Res. 2020;11(2):64.

156. On behalf of the Trail Network, Solomon JJ, Danoff SK, Goldberg HJ, Woodhead F, Kolb M, et al. The Design and Rationale of the Trail1 Trial: A Randomized Double-Blind Phase 2 Clinical Trial of Pirfenidone in Rheumatoid Arthritis-Associated Interstitial Lung Disease. Adv Ther. 2019 Nov;36(11):3279–87.

157. Bhaskar Sb. Clinical trial registration: A practical perspective. Indian J Anaesth. 2018;62(1):10.

158. Andrade C. Sample Size and its Importance in Research. Indian Journal of Psychological Medicine. 2020 Jan;42(1):102–3.

159. Suresh K. An overview of randomization techniques: An unbiased assessment of outcome in clinical research. J Hum Reprod Sci. 2011;4(1):8.

160. Getz KA, Wenger J, Campo RA, Seguine ES, Kaitin KI. Assessing the Impact of Protocol Design Changes on Clinical Trial Performance. American Journal of Therapeutics. 2008 Sep;15(5):450–7.
161. Krishnankutty B, Naveen Kumar B, Moodahadu L, Bellary S. Data management in clinical research: An overview. Indian J Pharmacol. 2012;44(2):168.
162. Yao B, Zhu L, Jiang Q, Xia H. Safety Monitoring in Clinical Trials. Pharmaceutics. 2013 Jan 17;5(4):94–106.
163. Varun Saharawat. Data Analysis Techniques in Research – Methods, Tools & Examples. 2024.
164. Munshi R, Pilliwar C, Maurya M. Public disclosure of clinical trial results at Clinical Trial Registry of India- need for transparency in research! Perspect Clin Res. 2023;14(2):81.

Chapter 5

THESIS WRITING

A thesis is the compass of academic inquiry.

5.1 Understanding the purpose of the thesis/ dissertation

A doctoral dissertation serves as an official defence of a certain thesis. "Substantial" and "original" are two important concepts when describing a dissertation. It is a methodical technique to study where a hypothesis is developed and evidence is gathered to confirm or refute it. A thesis is a large effort in which scholars gain and impart new knowledge. It is an attempt by a scholar to investigate, evaluate, and advance their field of study of choice. They choose a topic to study first (1). They then choose what it is they wish to learn. A thesis should provide a thoroughly researched and unique work, pique readers' interest, and add to the corpus of knowledge in a particular field of study. It serves several key purposes

a) **Research exploration**: A thesis allows a student or researcher to delve deeply into a specific topic or question within their academic discipline. It requires extensive research, critical analysis, and the synthesis of existing knowledge.

b) **Knowledge contribution**: A thesis should contribute to the field by proposing a new theory, presenting new empirical findings, or offering a fresh perspective on an existing topic. It adds to the overall understanding of the subject matter.

c) **Problem-solving**: Many theses are research-based and aim to address a specific research question or problem. They provide solutions, insights, or recommendations that can be valuable for addressing real-world issues.

d) **Skill development**: Composing a thesis is a challenging academic task requiring proficiency in analysis, creative thinking, research, and good communication. It frequently represents the high point of a student's academic career and demonstrates their capacity for independent research.

e) **Academic evaluation**: A thesis is often a requirement for completing a degree program, such as a master's or doctoral program. It assesses students' understanding of the subject matter and their ability to conduct scholarly research.

f) **Professional development**: These can be valuable for future career prospects. They demonstrate expertise in a specific area and can be a credential that opens opportunities in academia, research, or certain professions.

g) **Building on existing knowledge**: A thesis builds upon the existing body of knowledge in a field, helping future researchers and scholars to better understand and expand upon the topic.

5.2 Features of a successful thesis

A good thesis has the following qualities:

- A good thesis should be specific, clear, and focused.
- It must solve an existing problem in society, organization, government, and others.
- It should be contestable and propose an arguable point that people can agree with or disagree with.
- A good thesis does not use general terms and abstractions.
- A good thesis should be definable.
- It anticipates the counter-arguments.
- Clarity in language.

5.3 University guidelines for thesis writing

Every university has its guidelines when it comes to thesis writing. These regulations cover font size, alignment, layout, style, numbering, headings, footers, chapter parts, total number of pages, plagiarism criteria, and other features. Each university establishes its guidelines, which researchers must adhere to to ensure that their thesis satisfies all requirements (2,3). In India, most organizations work under the University Grant Commission (UGC) to approve students' post-graduation or PhD to represent a good thesis work; the thesis must be clear, definite, and have a logical structure according to a set pattern approved by the UGC. Any formal thesis writing must be presented, with special attention to the structure and look of the document. The first thing to remember is that you should only do your thesis work in the specified format. Adopting format consistency and closely adhering to the extra directions help the student more effectively convey their scholarly work (4).

5.4 Organization of Thesis Chapters

While each university may have unique guidelines, the sequence of chapters in a thesis is a universal language across institutions. This universality brings a sense of familiarity and ease in organizing your work. Based on extensive literature or university guidelines, we have suggested a thesis division, as mentioned below.

- Title page
- Certificates
- Index
- List of tables

- List of Figures
- Abbreviations
- Chapter separators
- Abstract
- Introduction
- Review of literature
- Aim, objective, rationale
- Plan of work
- Research methodology
- Results and discussion
- Conclusion
- Future prospective
- List of publications
- References
- Appendices
- Errata.

5.4.1 *Title page*

A thesis's title page should be eye-catching and establish the overall direction of the study. The name of the research scholar, the name of the guide, the registration number, the branch, the name of the institution, the address, and the year are all listed on this page. The primary focus of the title page is the title, which should be brief, intriguing, and educational so that readers can understand the nature of the research.

The list of required words for the title may differ depending on the requirements set forth by the university. It could have 100, 150, or more characters, etc. The research kind, the procedures/techniques employed, the formulation type, and any particular focus—such as a medication or medical condition—should all be briefly stated in the title. Readers choose whether or not to read based on what they see first. An appealing and interesting title increases readers' likelihood of interacting with the thesis. As a result, creating a compelling title is crucial to the thesis's success and grabbing readers' attention (5,6).

Computer-aided Drug Repurposing of NSAIDs and Local Anesthetics for Novel Therapeutic Use as Anticancer, Antibacterial, and Antifungal Agents.

Image 5.1: Example of title.

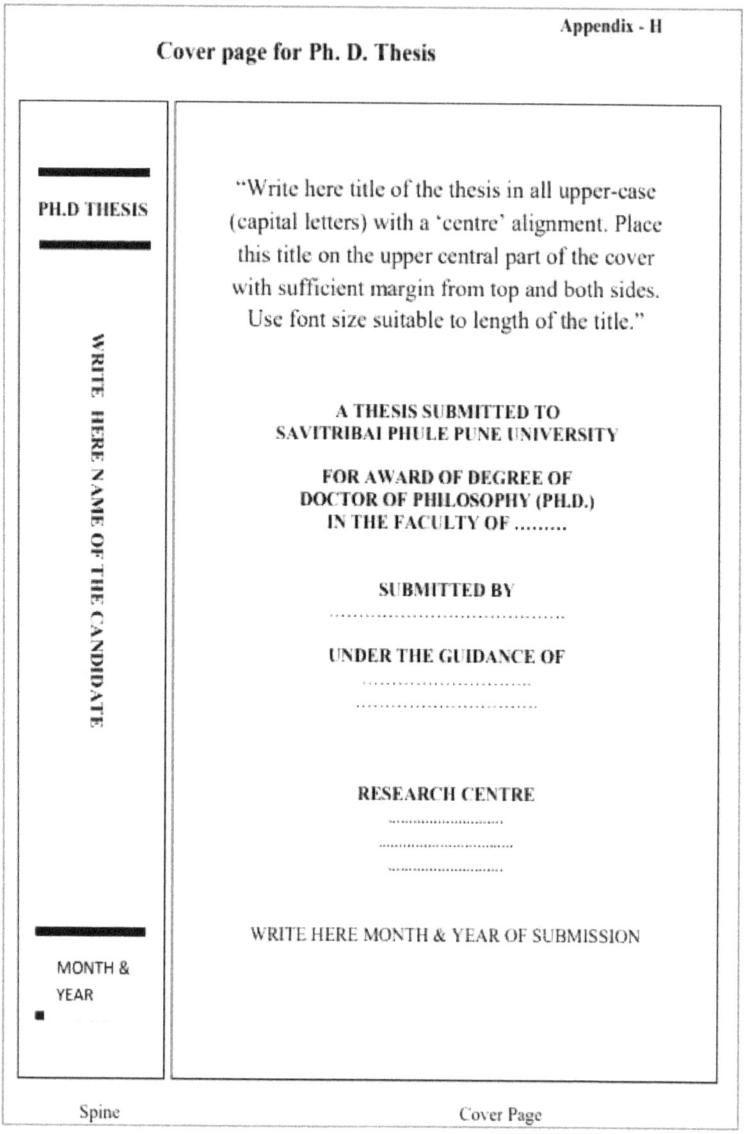

Appendix - H

Cover page for Ph. D. Thesis

PH.D THESIS

WRITE HERE NAME OF THE CANDIDATE

MONTH & YEAR

"Write here title of the thesis in all upper-case (capital letters) with a 'centre' alignment. Place this title on the upper central part of the cover with sufficient margin from top and both sides. Use font size suitable to length of the title."

A THESIS SUBMITTED TO
SAVITRIBAI PHULE PUNE UNIVERSITY

FOR AWARD OF DEGREE OF
DOCTOR OF PHILOSOPHY (PH.D.)
IN THE FACULTY OF ....

SUBMITTED BY
....

UNDER THE GUIDANCE OF
....
....

RESEARCH CENTRE
....
....
....

WRITE HERE MONTH & YEAR OF SUBMISSION

Spine

Cover Page

Image 5.2: Title/ cover page (7).

5.4.2   Certificates

Dissertations frequently call for a variety of certificates, per university policies. These credentials have several uses and are necessary for a PhD holder's research projects.

- ***Certificate of research scholar:*** This formally recognises completion of research tenure and validates commitment and contributions to scholarly activities.

- ***Certificate of the guide:*** A certificate confirming the guidance and supervision provided by the thesis director, supervisor, or guide, as well as the affiliation with the university.

- ***Declarations:*** A formal statement affirming the originality and integrity of the research work and ensuring adherence to academic honesty standards.

- ***Acknowledgement:*** An expression of gratitude toward individuals, staff, and institutions for their support and contribution to the research scholar's academic journey.

These certificates are required to ensure the integrity, legality, and acknowledgment of the research work conducted by PhD holders. Adhering to the university's guidelines and obtaining these certificates is essential for the completion and acceptance of the dissertation (8).

5.4.3   Index

A list of chapters, sections, subsections, and any other important headings or divisions, together with the corresponding page numbers, are usually included in an index. An index makes it easier for readers to find and browse the document and is required. It improves the document's readability and usability, making it easier for readers to locate pertinent information quickly. (9).

SR. NO.	CONTENT	PAGE NO.
.1	Introduction	1-20
2.	Literature review	21-25
3.	Aim, objectives and need of research	26
4.	Plan of research work	27
5.	Drug and material profile	28-31
6.	Research methodology	32-46
7.	Results and discussion	47-64
8.	Summary and conclusion	65-67
9.	References	68-73
10.	Plagiarism report	74
11.	Errata	75

Image 5.3: Example of the index page.

5.4.4   *List of tables and figures*

In a thesis, the list of tables and list of figures provides readers with easy access to all the tables and figures included in the document, along with their respective page numbers. This saves readers time by allowing them to quickly locate specific tables or figures without searching through the entire document. The inclusion of a list of tables and figures in a thesis significantly contributes to the document's overall structure, readability, and accessibility, thereby enhancing the reader's understanding and engagement with the research presented (10).

5.4.5   Abbreviations

Shorter versions of widely used terms are called acronyms. Shorter forms work better than longer ones regarding reducing word repetition in the thesis, reducing the likelihood of copying. The following is the meaning of abbreviations:

- Efficiency
- Clarity
- Consistency
- Ease of reference
- Professionalism.

5.4.6   Abstract

A summary of the complete study endeavor is given in the abstract. An abstract is essential for summarizing a thesis's main points, making a work easier to access, supporting decision-making, improving communication, increasing discoverability, and maintaining academic integrity among academics. The abstract's primary elements are the background, goal, methodology, key findings, discussion, closing thoughts, and future directions. After reading the abstract, readers will have no trouble comprehending the study's objectives, methods, and justifications. University requirements state that the abstract should not exceed 300–500 words. (11).

5.4.7   Chapter's separators

Chapter separators in a thesis are pages designed to separate different chapters or sections within the thesis visually. They enhance the overall look of the thesis and help readers easily navigate to specific chapters without spending time searching. These separators typically feature the chapter title in a prominent and visually appealing format. They are placed before the start of each new chapter or major section in the thesis. By incorporating chapter separators, the thesis achieves a more organized and professional appearance, making it easier for readers to locate and access relevant content (12).

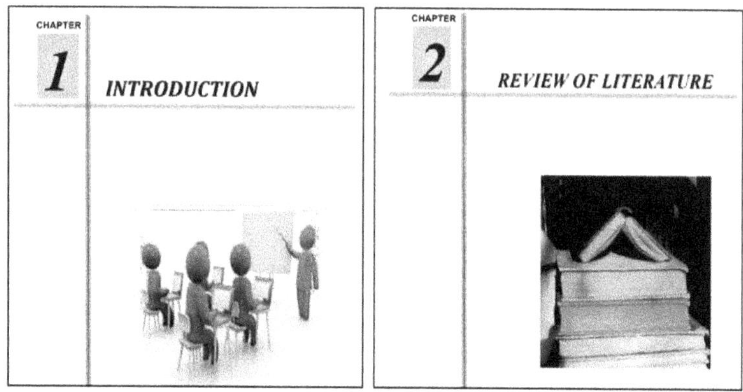

Image 5.4: Example of separators.

5.4.8   *Introduction*

The study's beginning and a summary of the research topic are provided in the introduction. It gives background information and could contain current events and worldwide data. The study's necessity is explained in the introduction, which also identifies its innovative features and outlines expectations for its findings (13).

How do you write an introduction part?

- **Capture the reader's interest**

You must first draw the reader in by outlining a more general theme connected to your research. To increase effect, draw on studies, information, quotes from governmental agencies, major writers on the subject, and international or national professional associations.

- **Give an overview of your research topic**

Your discussion should then begin by detailing the broader aspects of the topic before focusing on the specific topic of your research. When you do this, assuming that the reader knows nothing about your topic is a good idea. Therefore, definitions/terms, drawing on key research, and an overview of the methodology used need to be clarified and explained.

- **Detail on how your research is going to contribute**

You must then tell your idea for undertaking the research topic, demonstrating the main reasons why the research will significantly contribute to the current body of research. This can be achieved by demonstrating a gap or limitation with existing research and then showing how your research will resolve this.

- **Explain what your interest is in the topic**

You then have to explain why you chose the subject. These might be connected to your earlier studies, employment, or experiences.

- **List your research objectives**

You need to include your three or four overarching research objectives. Also, include corresponding research questions if the research is qualitative or hypotheses if it is quantitative. The former are usually derivatives of the research objectives. Note, though, that these objectives, questions, or hypotheses are fluid and can be tweaked as you undertake the research.

- **Give a forthcoming chapter overview**

The final part of the introduction provides an overview of the rest of the chapters in the thesis. The other sections can be in any order, provided it is a logical sequence (14).

5.4.9 Review of literature

A thesis's cornerstone is its literature review, which compiles a wide range of works on the subject of the study. This can be difficult to do because so much material is available from reputable sources and search engines. Examining prior research gives the study problem perspective and aids in researchers' comprehension of its importance and applicability in the larger academic debate. After being retrieved, the pertinent material on the chosen topic is organized orderly. Effective literature organization can be achieved by various strategies, including grouping the works according to publication year, results, titles, techniques, or conclusions. Every method presents an alternative viewpoint on the corpus of current knowledge, facilitating readers' comprehension of prior study findings and what gaps exist (15,16).

5.4.10 Aim, objective, rationale

Aim and objective are two crucial phrases in research that are sometimes used synonymously. But there's a basic distinction between the two. A research study's aim is its overarching goal or purpose, whereas its objectives are more detailed declarations outlining the procedures or activities required to reach the aim. Aim explains the purpose of the study and the goals the researcher has in mind. It offers a broad overview of the study's objectives and course. It also aids in providing a clear focus for the study and directing the research process. The objectives are more precise and quantifiable than the aim, offering a clear path forward for the study. Objectives help to clarify the research question, identify the key variables, and outline the research methodology. They are often used to break down the aim of the research into smaller, more manageable tasks. They help to provide structure and direction to the research and ensure that the researcher stays on track. They are often **S**pecific, **M**easurable, **A**chievable, **R**elevant, and **T**ime-bound (acronym: SMART). We have included an example to help you better understand the distinction between aims and objectives.

Example:

Aim: To investigate the relationship between physical activity and mental health.

Objectives:

- To review the existing literature on the relationship between physical activity and mental health.
- To collect data on a sample population's physical activity levels and mental health.
- To analyze the data to determine the relationship between physical activity and mental health.
- To draw conclusions and make recommendations based on the findings of the study (17).

The rationale for one's research is the justification for undertaking a given study. It states the reason(s) why a researcher chooses to focus on the topic in question, including the significance and gaps the research intends to fill. In short, it is an explanation that rationalizes the need for the study (18).

5.4.11　*Plan of work*

The work plan outlines the step-by-step approach and all the tasks that will be undertaken to complete the research project. It provides a detailed roadmap of the research journey, including the methods, experiments, data collection, analysis, and other activities involved in achieving the research objectives. It serves as a guide for the researcher, ensuring that the research is conducted systematically and efficiently (19).

5.4.12　*Drug and excipient profile*

In a Ph.D. thesis, if a drug is being used in the research, detailed information about its drug should be provided. This includes:

- Name of the drug/ excipient
- Chemical name
- Molecular weight (MW)
- Solubility
- Crystal structure
- Bonds present
- Ability to bind
- Active sites
- Other

If the researchers work on an herbal drug project, then he/she needs to mention a plant profile that includes:

- Taxonomy
- Description

- Habitat
- Geographical distribution
- Medicinal uses
- Photographs, illustrations
- Etc.

By including this information, readers can gain a comprehensive understanding of the drug being studied and its properties relevant to the research (20).

5.4.13 Research methodology

It is also called *experimentation, experimental work, materials and methods, methodology,* etc., depending on institutions' guidelines. In a PhD thesis, detailing this part used for the research is important This includes:

- List of the materials required for the research.
- Describe the materials from which they were sourced and if they were authenticated.
- Mentioning the required equipment, instruments, software, rat model (if any), or cell lines.
- Specifying the make and model of machines or equipment used for the research.
- It also describes the study type, formulation technique, data collection methods and tools, etc.

By providing this information, the thesis becomes more comprehensive and effective. It ensures transparency and allows readers to understand the research process clearly (21,22).

5.4.14 Results and discussion

The effectiveness of the research is assessed in the section on outcomes and discussion. They are occasionally written under different chapter headings. It offers a thorough, non-manipulated analysis of the favorable, unfavorable, or satisfactory outcomes. Results include a summary of the key findings, integrating quantitative and qualitative findings, results presented with the proper visual aids, and statistics for quantitative data. Nonetheless, the discussion highlights study limitations, compares findings with other research, and clarifies the significance of findings on research questions (15).

5.4.15 Conclusion

The Conclusion section of a thesis summarizes the key findings of the research or project based on the obtained results. This section provides closure to the thesis by highlighting the significance of the findings and their implications for the research aim. It offers insights into the overall impact of the research and may suggest future directions or areas for further investigation (23).

5.4.16 Future perspective

In the Future Prospects section, researchers discuss potential avenues for further research or innovation. It helps readers understand potential areas for exploration and encourages continued inquiry in the field. In the future prospects, researchers may contribute to the ongoing advancement of knowledge and inspire further research endeavors (24).

5.4.17   List of Publications

The List of Publications includes the researcher's own published works, such as reviews, research articles, conferences, chapters, or any other work. This section provides a quick reference to the researcher's contributions to the field and allows readers to access the publications easily (25).

5.4.18   References

You have to provide credit where credit is due when using someone else's work in your thesis. This is the purpose of citations. Citations make it clear where you got your knowledge, making it easier for others to follow your trail and validate your assertions. It's important to adhere to your university's norms regarding citing sources, as different universities may have different requirements. Your thesis is built upon references. They are the energy that propels your research trip; they are more than just a list of names and titles (26).

5.4.19   Appendices

These materials are placed in the appendices to provide additional detail and support for your thesis. Including such information can enhance the credibility and completeness of research. It includes:

- Participant Letters/Forms: informed consent/ CRF
- Surveys/Questionnaires
- Supplemental Tables/Figures/Graphs/Images
- Raw Data
- Permissions and Copyright certificate
- Plagiarism report

- Ethics committee approval letter
- Plant authentication certificate (27).

5.4.20 Errata

Correcting errors or inaccuracies found after the thesis has been published or submitted is the purpose of an errata in a thesis. Authors preserve the integrity of their work by admitting and correcting any mistakes that could have impacted the precision or dependability of their conclusions by publishing an erratum.

5.5 Originality Enhancement: Strategies for removing plagiarism

Presenting someone else's work as one's own is known as plagiarism. The presentation involves using it in copies or reproductions without crediting the original author. Phrases, clauses, sentences, paragraphs, or larger excerpts from published or unpublished work (including the Internet) beyond permissible collaboration are considered plagiarism if copied without citing the original author. There are two types of plagiarism: deliberate (dishonest plagiarism) and inadvertent (negligent plagiarism) (28). Presenting someone else's work as one's own is known as plagiarism. The presentation involves using it in copies or reproductions without giving credit to the original author. Phrases, clauses, sentences, paragraphs, or larger excerpts from published or unpublished work (including the Internet) that go beyond the bounds of permissible collaboration are considered plagiarism if they are copied without citing the original author. There are two types of plagiarism: deliberate (dishonest plagiarism) and inadvertent (negligent plagiarism) (28). Notably, the interpretation of this proportion may differ based on the particular standards issued by the newspaper or organization.

5.5.1   *Levels of Plagiarism*

Table 5.1: Level of plagiarism.

Level 0: Similarities up to 10%, minor similarities, no penalty
Level 1: Similarities above 10% to 40%
Level 2: Similarities above 40% to 60%
Level 3: Similarities above 60%.

This raised plagiarism may require revision or further investigation. Software such as Turnitin, Unicheck, Scribbr, Grammarly, PlagScan, Quetext, and Plagramme can be used to detect plagiarism. This software is either paid or unpaid. Addressing plagiarism after compiling your data is mandatory to ensure an impactful thesis. If high plagiarism percentages are detected, necessary revisions must be made to remove them and ensure originality in your work (29).

5.5.2   *Bonus tips to remove plagiarism*

- *Utilize paraphrasing tools:* To reword sentences and paragraphs while maintaining the original meaning, use online resources such as Quillbot.

- *Reframe using your own words:* Rather than directly copying sentences, restate the information in your own words. This eliminates plagiarism and demonstrates understanding and interpretation of the content.

- *Employ synonyms:* Replace specific words or phrases with synonyms to alter the structure and wording of the text while preserving the core message. This helps in maintaining originality while avoiding duplication.

- *Implement abbreviations*: Introduce abbreviations or acronyms for commonly used terms to add a unique touch to the text. However, ensure that the abbreviations are appropriate and understandable within the context.

- *Ensure proper citation*: Whenever referencing external sources or ideas, adhere to proper citation guidelines such as APA, MLA, or Chicago style. This acknowledges the original authorship and prevents plagiarism allegations.

5.6 Editing, formatting, and proofreading of thesis

Editing, formatting, and proofreading come last in the thesis writing process, following data compilation and plagiarism checks. Enhancing the content's logical flow, clarity, and organization is the main goal of editing, ensuring the reader understands the presented ideas. Formatting follows the particular style rules and criteria established by the magazine or academic institution. To ensure a polished and error-free final product, proofreading entails carefully reviewing the manuscript to fix typographical, grammatical, punctuation, and spelling issues. The general goal of thesis refining is to improve the thesis's overall caliber and professionalism so that it can be submitted and published in academic settings (30). The final stage is to submit to the appropriate university or institute after making all necessary adjustments and ensuring all rules are followed. This entails following the precise submission guidelines set forth by your organization and supplying all required paperwork for review and approval (31).

5.7 Common mistakes should be avoided during thesis writing and maintaining academic integrity

The common mistakes that can result in negative effects should be avoided during thesis writing, as mentioned in Table 5.2

Table 5.2: Common mistakes along with the consequences.

S. No	Common mistakes	Consequences
1	Lack of planning	Failing to create a detailed outline or timeline for a thesis can lead to disorganization and delays.
2	Poor research	Insufficient or outdated research can weaken the credibility of a thesis.
3	Inadequate editing	Neglecting thorough proofreading and editing may result in errors and unclear writing.
4	Ignoring feedback	Not seeking feedback from peers, advisors, or professors can lead to missed opportunities for improvement.
5	Plagiarism	Failing to properly cite sources or plagiarize content undermines academic integrity and credibility.
6	Overwhelming detail	Including unnecessary or excessive detail can obscure key points and confuse readers.
7	Procrastination	Waiting until the last minute to work on your thesis can result in a rush (32).

5.7.1 *How do you maintain academic integrity?*

- *Proper Citation:* Always give credit to original sources through accurate citation.

- *Avoid Plagiarism:* Use your own words and ideas, and properly attribute others' work.

- *Respect Copyright:* Obtain permission for copyright and adhere to fair use guidelines.

- *Data Integrity:* Ensure accuracy and transparency in data collection, analysis, and reporting.

- *Collaboration*: Collaborate ethically with colleagues and acknowledge their contributions.

- *Honesty:* Present your findings, interpretations, and conclusions honestly.

- *Peer Review:* Engage in peer review processes to ensure rigor and quality in academic work.

In conclusion, we can create an effective thesis by following best practices and avoiding typical blunders. A thesis that makes a significant contribution to the subject of study can be produced at a high standard by adhering to academic honesty, carrying out exhaustive research, and soliciting feedback (33).

5.8 References

1. Bitchener J, Banda M. Postgraduate Students' Understanding of the Functions of Thesis Sub-genres: The Case of the Literature Review.
2. Bartha, Tibor. Guidelines to Thesis Writing. University Of Veterinary Medicine Budapest; 2016.
3. Abdel-Magid. Guidelines for Thesis Preparation. 2014.
4. Catherine bitker rochester. Ugc PHD Thesis Guidelines. 2024.
5. Glatthorn, Allan A., and Randy L. Joyner. Writing the winning thesis or dissertation: A step-by-step guide. Corwin Press; 2005.
6. OCollins, G. A Short Guide to Writing a Thesis. ATF Press; 2011.
7. Savitribai Phule Pune University (Formerly University of Pune) CIRCULAR NO. 14/2OI7.
8. Rawlins, P.L.C. Students' perceptions of the formative potential of the National Certificate of Educational Achievement: a thesis presented in partial fulfillment of the requirements of the degree of PhD in Education. Massey University; 2007.
9. Viharos, Zsolt János. Thesis Of Phd Dissertation.
10. Ildikó, K. and József, T. Theses of Doctoral (PhD) Dissertation.
11. Zecevic, Svetlana. PhD Thesis Abstract.
12. David S. How to complete and survive a doctoral dissertation. St. Martin's Griffin; 2014.
13. Leshem, Shosh, Eli Bitzer, and Vernon Trafford. Writing the Introduction Chapter of PhD Theses. Vol. 12. 163-175; 2018.
14. Hill J, Sleep B, Drake J, Fryer M. The Effect of Intraparticle Porosity and Interparticle Voids on the Hydraulic Properties of Soilless Media. Vadose Zone Journal. 2019 Jan;18(1):1–13.
15. Faryadi Q. PhD Thesis Writing Process: A Systematic Approach—How to Write Your Literature Review. CE. 2018;09(16):2912–9.
16. Ridley, Diana. The Literature Review: A Step-by-Step Guide for Students. SAGE Study Skills Series; 2012. 232 p.
17. Difference between the Aim and Objectives of a Research Study. ScholarHangout. 2023;
18. Hambrick R. The Identity, Purpose, and Future of Doctoral Education. Journal of Public Administration Education. 1997 May;3(2):133–48.
19. Korrapati, Raghu. Five-Chapter Model for Research Thesis Writing: 108 Practical Lessons for MS/MBA/M. Tech/M. Phil/LLM/Ph. D Students. In: Modern pharmaceutics. Diamond Pocket Books Pvt Ltd; 2002.

20. Banker, Gilbert S., Juergen Siepmann, and Christopher Rhodes (last). Modern pharmaceutics. CRC Press; 2002.
21. Pemberton CLA. A "How-to" Guide for the Education Thesis/Dissertation Process. Kappa Delta Pi Record. 2012 Apr 30;48(2):82–6.
22. Andrews, Richard, and Jude England. New forms of dissertation. In: The SAGE handbook of digital dissertations and theses. 2012. p. 31–46.
23. Bunton D. The structure of PhD conclusion chapters. Journal of English for Academic Purposes. 2005 Jul;4(3):207–24.
24. Nuttin, Joseph. Future time perspective and motivation: Theory and research method. Psychology Press; 2014.
25. Energy, Hydrogen. An Investigation on Advanced Functional Carbonaceous Materials for High-Performance Composites in Fuel Cell Applications. In: List of Publications Journal papers (Thesis). 2023. p. 182.
26. Azadeh F, Vaez R. The accuracy of references in P h D theses: a case study. Health Info Libraries J. 2013 Sep;30(3):232–40.
27. Thompson P. Literature Reviews in Applied PhD Theses: Evidence and Problems. In: Hyland K, Diani G, editors. Academic Evaluation [Internet]. London: Palgrave Macmillan UK; 2009 [cited 2024 Mar 21]. p. 50–67. Available from: http://link.springer.com/10.1057/9780230244290_4
28. Plagiarism Policy of the University of Pune.
29. Lancaster, T. Effective and efficient plagiarism detection. London South Bank University; 2003.
30. Singh, B. P. Preventing the plagiarism in the digital age with special reference to Indian Universities. International Journal of Information Dissemination and Technology. 2016;6(4):281–7.
31. Harwood, N. Proofreading and Editing in Student and Research Publication Contexts: International Perspectives. Taylor & Francis Group. 2024;
32. Levin M. Academic integrity in action research. Action Research. 2012 Jun;10(2):133–49.
33. Rotbamrung, Wanida, and Monthon Kanokpermpoon. Rhetorical structure analysis on a results-discussion chapter by Thai postgraduate students. Thammasat University; 2022.

Chapter 6

IMAGE CREATION

Images speak louder than words.

6.1 Overview

The process of conveying information, concepts, or data through visual aids such as maps, diagrams, charts, graphs, photographs, and illustrations is called "visual representation". These visual aids are meant to help the viewer understand the material; they often replace or enhance written descriptions (1).

6.2 Why does an attractive image, graphs, graphical abstract, etc. need to be created?

It includes the following reasons:

- Improved comprehension: Visual aids make difficult concepts easier to understand.
- Readers are drawn in and kept interested by visuals.
- Skillfully created graphics convey the caliber and expertise of the study.
- Visuals make information more accessible to diverse audiences, including those with different learning styles.
- Impact: Eye-catching images create a lasting impression that highlights the importance of the study. (2).

Benefits of own-created visual elements

a) **Authenticity:** You can ensure that your pictures are original and work by making them yourself. This gives the research more legitimacy and authenticity.

b) **Clarity and precision:** You can tailor your visuals to precisely convey the information you want to communicate (3).

c) **Customization:** This lets you alter them to fit your unique needs and preferences, which improves the overall presentation of your thesis.

d) **Illustration of concepts:** Some ideas or conclusions could be complicated and challenging to convey in words alone. You can more effectively show these ideas and help your audience understand them by using your own generated diagrams, graphs, and photos (4).

e) **Intellectual property rights**: By creating your visuals, retain full control over their usage and distribution. This can be particularly important if plan to publish your thesis or use excerpts from it in other works.

In the following part, we've introduced some fundamental tools and applications for image design.

6.3 Software and tools for better visual representations

6.3.1 Microsoft PowerPoint

With its many image preparation features, users may improve, alter, and personalize photos to produce visually appealing presentations.

It is used for:

a) **Inserting images**: You can insert images into your slides by selecting the "Insert" tab and then choosing "Pictures" to select an image file from your computer or "Online Pictures" to search for images online (5).

b) **Editing images**: PowerPoint provides basic editing tools like crop, resize, rotate, and adjust brightness/contrast.

c) **Image styles and effects**: It offers various pre-designed styles and effects to apply to your images, such as shadows, reflections, and 3D effects (6).

d) **Image corrections**: You can adjust the colour, sharpness, and other aspects of an image using the "Corrections" options under the "Format Picture" pane. This allows you to fine-tune the appearance of your images to better suit your presentation (7).

e) **Image cropping and masking**: PowerPoint lets you crop images to focus on specific areas or remove unwanted parts.

f) **Background removal**: PowerPoint includes a feature called "Remove Background" which allows you to easily remove the background from an image to isolate the subject. This feature can be found under the "Format Picture" pane.

g) **Image compression**: PowerPoint has options for picture compression that might help you save the file size of your presentation. To maximize file size without noticeably lowering quality, you can apply compression to each image separately or to every image in the presentation (8).

These are but a handful of Microsoft PowerPoint's image preparation tools. The PowerPoint image that was produced is shown below.

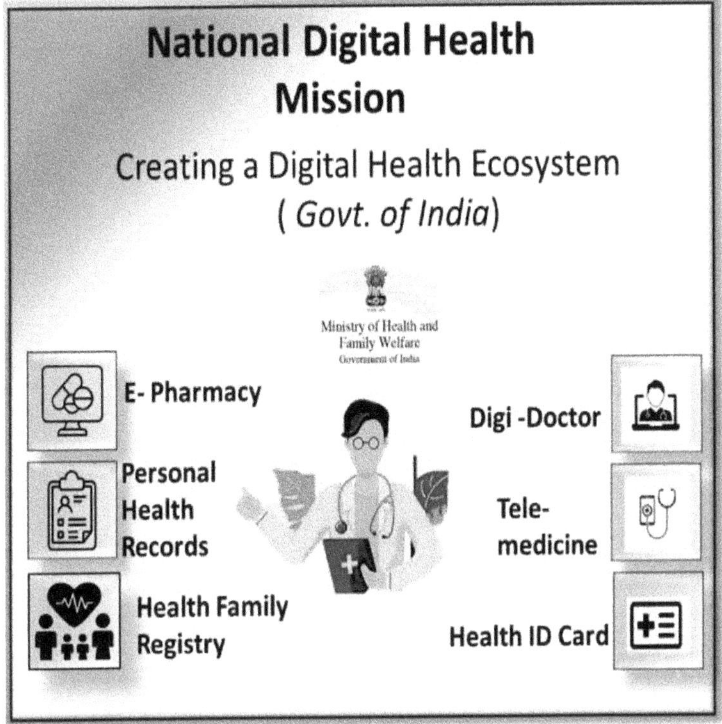

Image 6.1: National digital health mission.

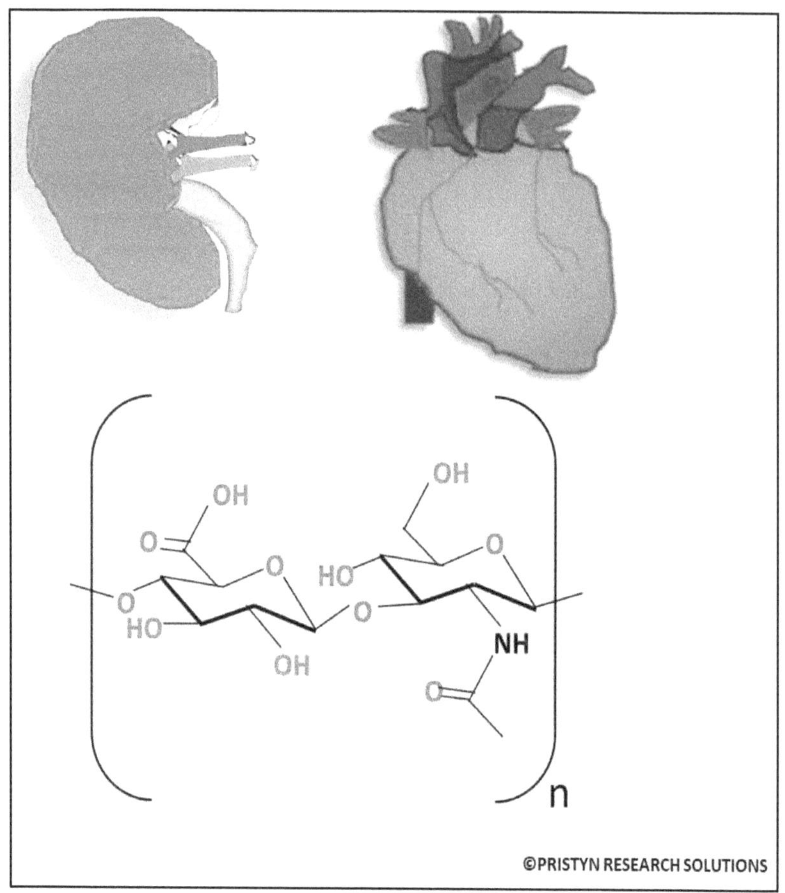

Image 6.2: Structure and figures.

6.3.2 *Inkscape*

Inkscape is a well-known open-source vector graphics editor for producing and modifying vector graphics, including illustrations, diagrams, logos, icons, and other visual elements. It has many features and tools comparable to those found in commercial vector graphics programs like Adobe Illustrator (9).

Key features of Inkscape

- **Vector graphics editing**: Create and edit scalable vector graphics.
- **Drawing tools**: Various shapes, lines, and freehand drawing tools.
- **Object manipulation**: Move, resize, rotate, and group objects easily.
- **Text support**: Format and stylize text within your designs.
- **Color and fill effects**: Apply colors, gradients, patterns, and transparency.
- **Path operations**: Combine, subtract, and manipulate shapes and paths.
- **Filters and effects**: Apply filters and effects to enhance your artwork.
- **Import and export**: Support for various file formats for compatibility.
- **Extensions and scripting**: Extend functionality through scripting and extensions.

6.3.3   *Microsoft Bing*

Microsoft Bing is a web search engine that facilitates rapid and effective information discovery online. Using AI, Image Creator from Designer allows you to create text-based images. It offers maps, photos, videos, search results, and more (10).

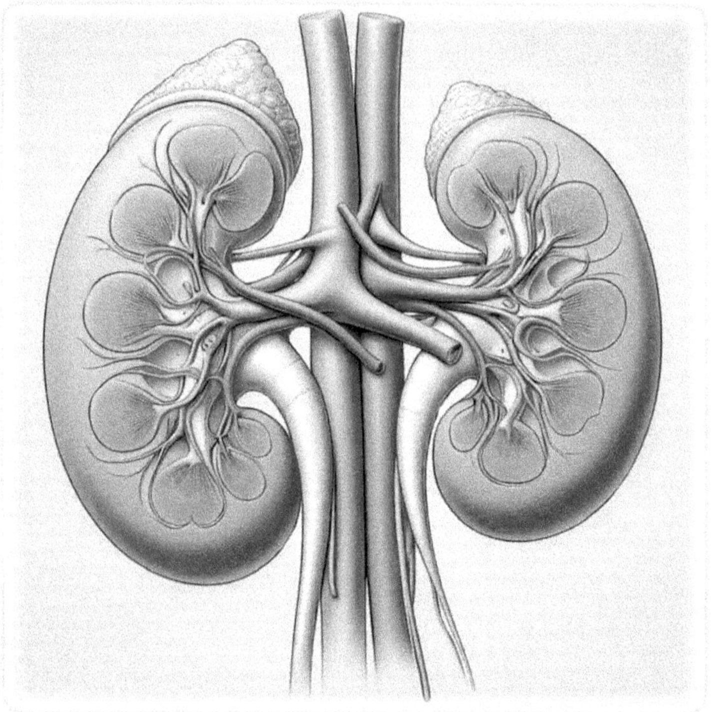

Images 6.3: Microsoft Bing's design.

6.3.4   Illustrator

Adobe Inc. is the firm behind Adobe Illustrator, a vector graphics editor. To produce a wide range of digital artwork, illustrations, logos, icons, typography, and intricate vector graphics, designers, artists, illustrators, and other creative professionals frequently utilize it. A flexible graphics editor that makes it possible to produce excellent illustrations, graphical abstracts, and infographics. It is comparable to Inkscape but has a subscription model (11).

6.3.5   *Biorender.com*

An AI-powered tool used for creating professional scientific illustrations and diagrams. It simplifies complex biological concepts (12).

a) **Scientific illustrations**: BioRender offers a sizable collection of scientifically correct icons, pictures, and templates covering biology, chemistry, medicine, and biotechnology. For projects, users may quickly search for certain symbols or browse through categories to find images that fit the bill.

b) **Graphical abstracts**: Researchers can create visually appealing graphical abstracts using BioRender's templates and tools. Graphical abstracts help summarize research findings and attract attention to scientific publications.

c) **Customization tools**: It offers modification options so users can change the icons' colors, sizes, forms, and styles to suit their requirements. Users can add annotations, text, arrows, and labels to their diagrams.

These AI tools and software allow users to create their diagrams easily. These tools are valuable not only for thesis writing but also for many other aspects of one's career. They save my time and effort. At last, these tools offer more efficient features for drawing images, graphs, and graphical abstracts, making them essential for visual content creation (13).

6.4 References

1. Bobek E, Tversky B. Creating visual explanations improves learning. Cogn Res Princ Implic. 2016;1(1):27.
2. Haeberli P. Paint by numbers: abstract image representations. In: Proceedings of the 17th annual conference on Computer graphics and interactive techniques [Internet]. Dallas TX USA: ACM; 1990 [cited 2024 Apr 10]. p. 207–14. Available from: https://dl.acm.org/doi/10.1145/97879.97902
3. McLean D. Adobe Photoshop and Illustrator techniques. Journal of Audiovisual Media in Medicine. 2002 Jan;25(2):79–81.
4. Rüger, S. How to write a good PhD thesis and survive the viva. The Open University; 2016.
5. Bothell, L. J. Microsoft® PowerPoint®. Business Technology Essentials. 2023;
6. Microsoft PowerPoint. University of Michigan Library. 2023;
7. Fletcher K. Adobe Presenter, Microsoft PowerPoint, and Blackboard Vista: tools that work together for creating and presenting online instructional content. In: Proceedings of the 37th annual ACM SIGUCCS fall conference: communication and collaboration [Internet]. St. Louis Missouri USA: ACM; 2009 [cited 2024 Apr 10]. p. 243–8. Available from: https://dl.acm.org/doi/10.1145/1629501.1629545
8. Tiwari RK, Sahoo G. Microsoft PowerPoint Files: A Secure Steganographic Carrier. International Journal of Digital Crime and Forensics. 2011 Oct 1;3(4):16–28.
9. Inkscape Overview. Available from: https://inkscape.org/about/
10. Eliceiri KW, Berthold MR, Goldberg IG, Ibáñez L, Manjunath BS, Martone ME, et al. biological imaging software tools. Nat Methods. 2012 Jul;9(7):697–710.
11. Adobe Illustrator. 2021; Available from Adobe. com
12. Kherlopian AR, Song T, Duan Q, Neimark MA, Po MJ, Gohagan JK, et al. A review of imaging techniques for systems biology. BMC Syst Biol. 2008 Dec;2(1):74.
13. Cetinic E, She J. Understanding and Creating Art with AI: Review and Outlook. ACM Trans Multimedia Comput Commun Appl. 2022 May 31;18(2):1–22.

Chapter 7

SOFTWARE & TOOLS

In the realm of software and AI, imagination is the only limit.

7.1 Overview

Software refers to a collection of programs, instructions, and data that enable a computer to perform specific tasks or functions (1). It includes the underlying systems and utilities that control hardware resources and permit program execution, as well as the applications that user's interface with directly, like word processors, web browsers, and video editors. Software is essential to many facets of research, analysis, teamwork, and communication in PhD programs. PhD candidates frequently have to conduct statistical studies, validate huge datasets, and present their results visually (2). They use software like Zotero, Mendeley, and EndNote to help them organize research papers, annotate documents, and manage citations effectively (3). Any document about the study is written using simple software, such as Microsoft Office. Experimental science uses software to plan experiments, gather data, and operate lab equipment. Additionally, the software provides several benefits, including automation, adaptability, efficacy, data security, and creativity. The software improves research productivity, precision, and dependability in PhD programs, empowering students to take on challenging assignments and share their discoveries with a wider academic audience.

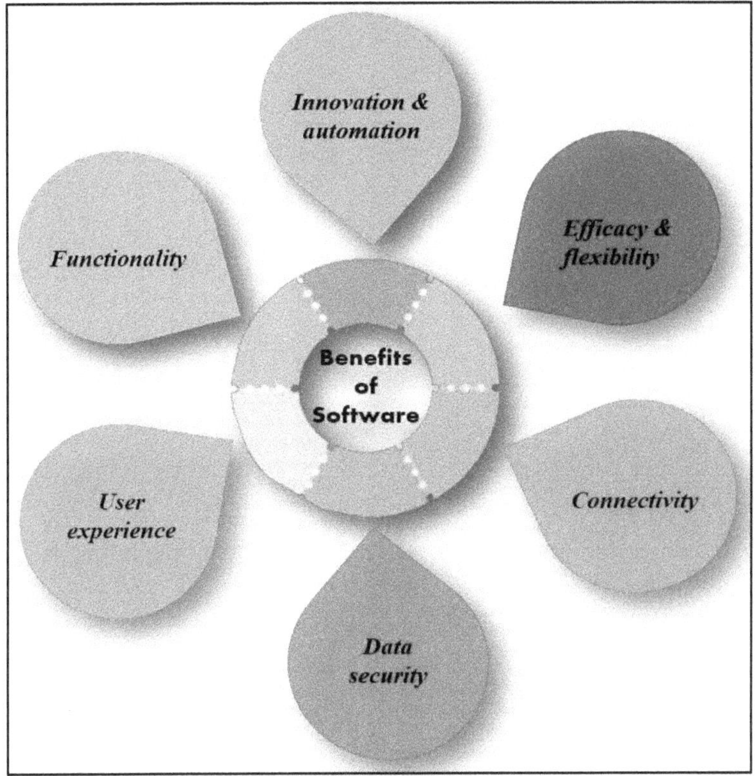

Image 7.1: Benefits of software.

7.2 Basic software

7.2.1   Benefits of using MS Office in academic or PhD writing

Microsoft (MS) Office software was developed by Microsoft in 1988 and is available in 35 different languages. It includes Word, Excel, and PowerPoint and is widely used and familiar to most researchers and students. Its ubiquity ensures easy access and compatibility across different devices and operating systems.

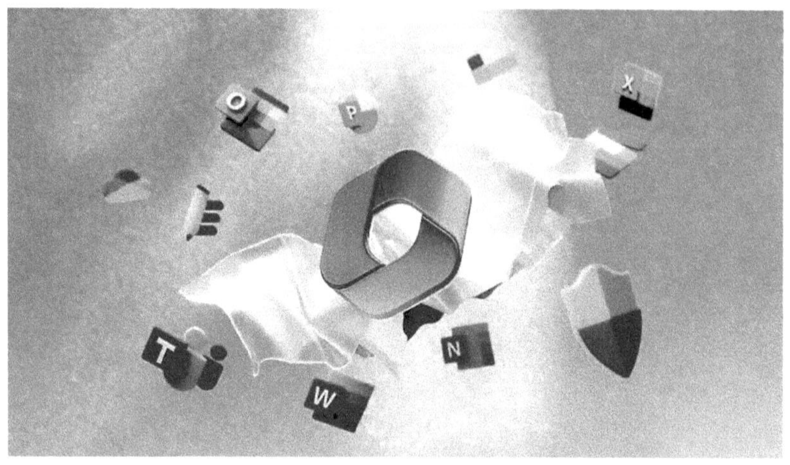

Image 7.2: Office applications
(https://www.aztechit.co.uk/blog/microsoft-office-365-benefits).

For research work and academic writing, Microsoft Word offers several advantages. It has formatting options, sharing and collaboration capabilities, citation and reference features, templates, auto-save, grammar and spelling checks, and easy access. All of these features make it user-friendly. It supports the upkeep of an orderly and consistent document flow (4). Microsoft Excel is useful for organizing and analyzing data and creating tables, charts, and graphs for visual representation. Researchers can use Excel to manage experimental data, perform statistical analysis, and generate graphical illustrations for publications (5). Teaching materials, conference posters, and academic presentations are frequently created using Microsoft PowerPoint. It is appropriate for successfully communicating research findings and concepts thanks to its user-friendly interface, slide templates, and multimedia integration capabilities (6). The Microsoft Office suite easily connects with other productivity services and tools, including Teams for online meetings and collaboration, OneNote for taking notes, and Outlook for email correspondence. This harmonious ecosystem increases productivity and workflow efficiency. Using Microsoft Office for academic or PhD writing allows for ease, effectiveness, and variety, enabling students and researchers to efficiently manage their records, information, and presentations as they work on their studies.

7.3 Frequently used software in academic writing
7.3.1   ChemDraw

ChemDraw is a versatile molecular sketching tool used by chemists and biologists to create professional, easy-to-understand figures of molecules for presentations or publications. This software also allows users to sketch reaction schemes and chemical drawings beyond molecular structures with precision and ease, so they can be moved into other programs, like MS Word, PowerPoint, and Adobe Illustrator (7).

ChemDraw offers several benefits

- Easy-to-use
- Customizable
- Include stereochemistry
- High-quality graphics and illustrations
- Integration with external chemistry databases.

The version of ChemDraw available to students and faculty varies depending on the institution. For example, UW-Eau Claire has a site license to ChemDraw Prime, which allows any student or faculty member to download a free copy of the application and install it on their personal computer (8).

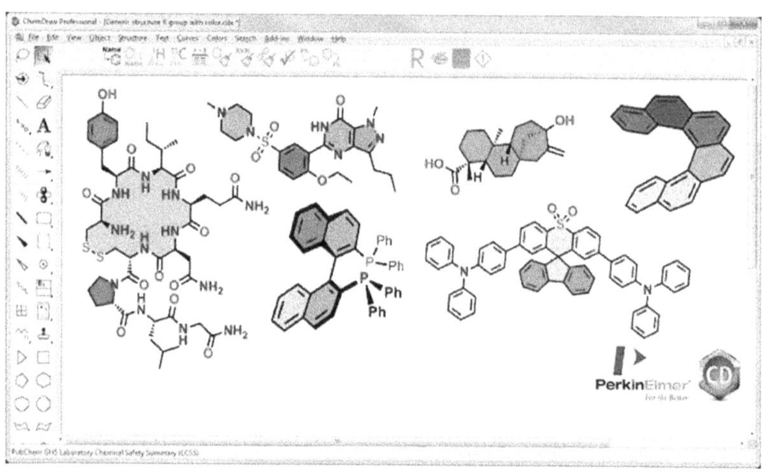

Image 7.3: Interface of ChemDraw.

Table 7.1: Summary of ChemDraw.

1.	Description	ChemDraw is a molecular drawing and visualization software.
2	Developer(s)	PerkinElmer Informatics, a division of PerkinElmer, Inc.
3	Initial Release	1985
4	Latest Version	23.0 / February 14, 2024
5	Alternative tools	MarvinSketch, ACD/ChemSketch, ChemDoodle, JChemPaint, Biovia Draw, etc.

7.3.2   Zotero

Scholars may better gather, arrange, and reference their materials for scholarly work using the reference management tool Zotero. Users can build customized libraries, integrate bibliographic material from websites, online databases, and PDFs, and produce citations and bibliographies in various citation formats. With Zotero, referencing is more accurate and efficient, and sources in academic papers are properly attributed. With Zotero, users can arrange their work to conform to any style guide or publication because it supports more than 10,000 citation styles. Citations can be imported and exported in formats like BibTeX, RefWorks, and Wikipedia Citation Templates. Users of Zotero can also design their unique citation styles (9).

Table7.2: Summary of Zotero

1.	**Description**	**It manages bibliographic data and related research materials, such as PDF and ePUB files.**
2	Developer(s)	Initially by the Center for History and New Media at George Mason University, now developed by the Corporation for Digital Scholarship.
3	Initial Release	October 5, 2006
4	Latest Version	6.0.30, released on November 2, 2023
5	Alternative tools	Mendeley, EndNote, RefWorks, Bib Tex, etc.

7.3.3   Quillbot

An AI-powered paraphrase tool called QuillBot is intended to assist writers in rephrasing sentences to increase the coherence and clarity of their work. It uses machine learning algorithms to scan text for synonyms and alternate wordings, which helps researchers write better, avoid plagiarism, and communicate ideas more clearly. It is an invaluable tool for academics who want to increase the quality of their writing and research because of its AI-powered capabilities, customizable choices, and ease of use. To increase clarity and elevate the caliber of their writing, alter the tone of their material (10).

Table7.3: Summary of Quillbot

1.	Description	AI-powered paraphrasing tool designed to assist writers in rephrasing sentences and improving the clarity and coherence of their writing.
2	Developer(s)	QuillBot LLC
3	Initial Release	-
4	Latest Version	Continuous updates and improvements
5	Alternative tools	Paraphrase Online, Spinbot, and SmallSEO Tools, etc.

7.3.4   *Turnitin*

Plagiarism is a serious issue in academic writing, including theses and publications. It involves using someone else's work, ideas, or words without proper citation or attribution. It is considered unethical and can lead to severe consequences, including academic penalties and damage to one's reputation (11). Academic institutions commonly utilize Turnitin, a plagiarism detection tool, to evaluate how unique students' writing is. It looks for possible plagiarism or incorrect citation instances by comparing submitted papers to a sizable database of scholarly and internet sources. Turnitin upholds high standards of scholarly conduct and ethical writing practices, assisting instructors and students in promoting academic integrity (12).

Table 7.4: Summary of Turnitin

1.	Description	**It is a web-based plagiarism detection service that compares submitted documents against a vast database of academic and online sources to identify potential instances of plagiarism or improper citation.**
2	Developer(s)	Turnitin LLC, a subsidiary of Advance Publications, Inc.
3	Initial Release	1997 by iParadigms, LLC, which later became Turnitin LLC.
4	Latest Version	Turnitin Feedback Studio
5	Alternative tools	Grammarly, Copyscape, Unicheck, PlagScan

7.3.5   *Grammarly*

Grammarly is an AI-powered writing tool that provides feedback on syntax, punctuation, style, tone, and clarity to help users write better. It gives users immediate feedback while they type, pointing up mistakes and offering suggestions for improvements to improve the caliber and readability of their writing. Grammarly offers a smooth platform and device integration and is accessible as a desktop, mobile, browser extension, and web application (13).

Table 7.5: Summary of Grammarly

1.	Description	**Grammar correction and suggestion tool.**
2	Developer(s)	Grammarly, Inc., an American technology company headquartered in San Francisco, California, develops and maintains the Grammarly writing assistant.
3	Initial Release	-
4	Latest Version	Continuous updates and improvements.
5	Alternative tools	ProWritingAid, Hemingway Editor, and WhiteSmoke, etc.

7.4 Statistical software

Statistical software is used for several purposes in data analysis, including quantitative data analysis, predictive modeling, text analysis, visualization, and data management. These tools are used in various industries, such as market research, education, healthcare, and business analytics. An ANOVA, regression analysis, descriptive analysis, chi-tests, and t-tests are the statistical tests done using this software.

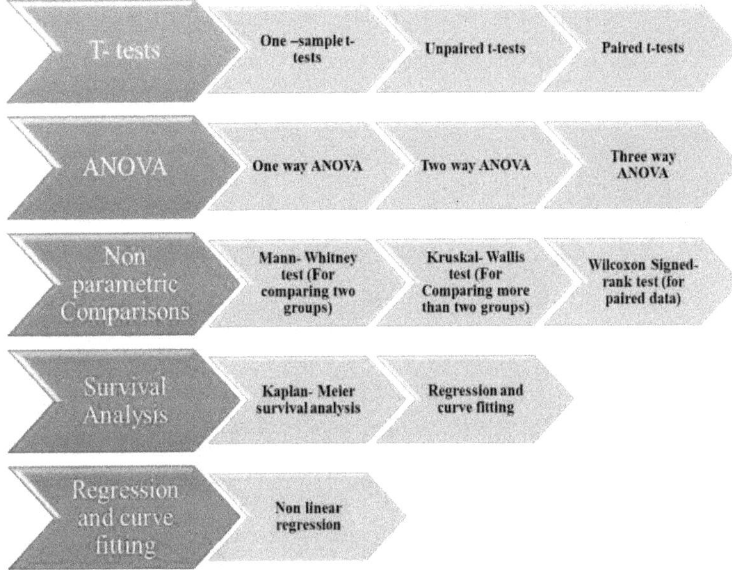

Image 7.4: Statistical test (14).

Statistical software plays an important role in the pharmaceutical field

- *Efficiency in Data Analysis:* Pharmaceutical experts can quickly and accurately provide results by using statistical software programs to analyze large datasets rapidly, perform statistical tests, and present data.

- *Compliance with Quality Guidelines:* These software packages help ensure compliance with quality guidelines such as Design of Experiment (DOE), Failure Modes and Effects Analysis (FMEA), and Statistical Process Control (SPC) outlined by regulatory bodies like the ICH, enhancing the quality and safety of pharmaceutical products (15).

- *Enhanced Decision-Making:* Pharmaceutical businesses can improve their decision-making processes and streamline operations using statistical tools to help them make well-informed judgments on population targeting, clinical trials, drug development, and market circumstances.

- *Accelerated Drug Discovery:* Statistical methods and predictive analytics in this software package aid in accelerating drug discovery processes by allowing researchers to analyze vast amounts of data, identify potential drugs faster, and focus on the most promising hypotheses, ultimately speeding up the drug development timeline (9).

- *Personalized Medicine Development:* Statistical software facilitates the integration of genomic sequencing, patient data, and electronic health records, enabling pharmaceutical companies to personalize medications based on individual genetic makeup. This leads to more effective and targeted treatments for patients.

- *Cost Reduction and Efficiency*: Pharmaceutical businesses can save costs by using data analytics to optimize medication development processes, minimize errors, enhance population health, and boost drug utilization efficiency. This will ultimately result in cost savings and better financial planning (16).

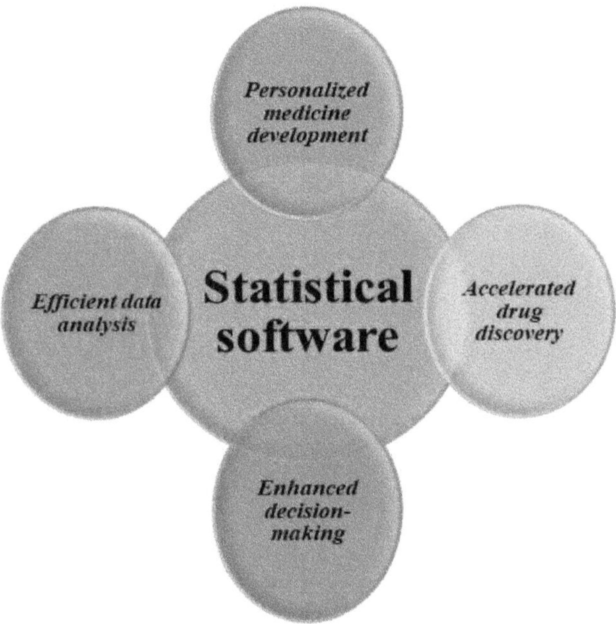

Image 7.5: Benefits of statistical software.

7.4.1   MS Excel

A flexible application, Microsoft Excel provides a range of statistical algorithms and data analysis capabilities. It's employed for:

- **Descriptive statistics**: Calculating basic descriptive statistics, such as mean, median, mode, standard deviation, variance, and quartiles.
- **Data visualization**: Excel's charting capabilities allow users to produce various graphs and charts, such as scatter plots, bar charts, line graphs, and histograms.
- **Regression analysis**: Excel has functions for carrying out linear regression analysis. This enables users to evaluate the

relationship between two variables and fit a straight line to their data. In addition, users can compute R-squared values and regression coefficients and forecast using the regression model.

- **Hypothesis testing**: Excel provides functions for conducting hypothesis tests, such as t-tests, chi-square tests, and F-tests. These tests allow users to assess the statistical significance of differences between groups or the association between variables.

- **ANOVA (Analysis of Variance)**: Excel includes functions for performing analysis of variance, which is used to compare means across multiple groups. ANOVA tests help users determine whether there are statistically significant differences between the group means.

- **Correlation analysis:** Correlation coefficients can be calculated with Excel using functions like Pearson's correlation coefficient and Spearman's rank correlation coefficient. These coefficients measure the intensity and direction of the association between two variables.

- **Pivot tables and pivot charts**: Excel's PivotTable and PivotChart functions let users easily summarize and examine big datasets. With PivotTables and PivotCharts, users can quickly aggregate data, compute summary statistics, and produce interactive representations (17).

Limitations: Excel has limitations in handling large datasets and performing complex statistical analyses. It may not be suitable for advanced statistical modeling or research-level analyses (18).

7.4.2 *Statistical Analysis System (SAS)*

SAS is a statistical software suite developed by the SAS Institute for data management, advanced analytics, multivariate analysis, business intelligence, criminal investigation, and predictive analytics (19).

- SAS began growing in 1966 and lasted until 1976 when it was co-founded by James Goodnight, Anthony Barr, Jane T. Helwig, and John Sall.
- SAS grew to be more inclusive during the 1980s and 1990s, with the implementation of new statistical techniques and additional components (20).

  SAS offers:

- Descriptive Statistics
- Hypothesis Testing (t-tests, ANOVA, chi-square tests)
- Regression Analysis (linear, logistic, Poisson)
- Survival Analysis
- Time Series Analysis
- Cluster Analysis
- Factor Analysis
- Multivariate Analysis
- Machine Learning Algorithms (decision trees, random forests, neural networks), etc.

Importance of SAS in the pharmaceutical sector

- Clinical Trials Analysis
- Drug Development
- Regulatory Compliance
- Drug Safety Monitoring

- Real-world Evidence Generation
- Predictive Analytics
- Personalized Medicine (21).

7.4.3   *Statistical package for the social sciences (spss)*

SPSS is a software package used for statistical analysis and data management. It is widely used in various industries to analyze and interpret complex data. SPSS allows for a variety of statistical analyses, including descriptive statistics, hypothesis testing (such as t-tests and ANOVA), regression analysis, factor analysis, cluster analysis, survival analysis, time series analysis, nonparametric statistics, and data visualization (22).

- SPSS's ability to analyze complex data, identify trends, patterns, and relationships, and make informed decisions based on the results is essential in the pharmaceutical sector.
- SPSS supports both analysis and modification of many kinds of data and almost all formats of structured data, including spreadsheets, plain text files, and relational databases such as SQL, SATA, and SAS (23).

Importance of SPSS in the pharmaceutical sector

1. Drug discovery
2. In clinical trials
3. In market research
4. Quality control
5. Pharmacovigilance (24).

7.4.4   *Stata (Statistics and Data)*

Stata is a useful tool for researchers and statisticians to analyze complex data sets because of its versatility, user-friendliness, and extensive statistical techniques. Stata is a critical tool used by researchers in the pharmaceutical industry to analyze preclinical and clinical study data from clinical trials. This data analysis helps researchers identify trends, patterns, and relationships in the data, which is important for making informed decisions in drug development, safety monitoring, and regulatory compliance. Researchers can then interpret the results and make decisions based on the findings (25).

Stata is used in the pharmaceutical sector for various purposes, including

1.   Data Visualization
2.   Predictive Modeling
3.   Data Management
4.   Statistical Analysis

7.4.5   *GraphPad Prism*

GraphPad Prism is a comprehensive program for curve fitting, scientific graphing, and biostatistics. Scientists, researchers, and professionals from various professions use it extensively, including top universities, hospitals, research facilities, and pharmaceutical businesses. The software has an easy-to-use interface that walks users through each analysis, providing help when needed and effectively recording and organizing work.

Key features of GraphPad prism:

- Wide range of statistical analyses: The software offers an extensive library of statistical analyses, including t-tests, ANOVA, regression, and survival analysis, which cater to the needs of researchers in various scientific disciplines (26).

- Streamlined data organization: GraphPad Prism is designed to facilitate the entry and organization of data for specific analyses. It supports quantitative and categorical data and provides structured tables tailored to different data types.

- Real-time updates and automation: The software automatically updates graphs and results in real time as changes are made to the data. Users can easily modify data, correct errors, or adjust analysis choices and instantly see updated results. The software also offers automation features, such as one-click regression analysis (27).

- Customizable graphs and data visualization: GraphPad Prism offers various customization options for graphs and data visualization.

- Integration with Other Programs: GraphPad Prism can import results, making it easier to integrate with other programs and systems (28).

GraphPad Prism has been developed by FDA rule 21 CFR Part 11, which pertains to businesses that submit experimental data to the FDA for clearance. However, as the FDA views GraphPad Prism as "off-the-shelf software," the user must adhere to these standards (29).

7.5 Drug design software

In biotechnology and pharmaceuticals, drug design software may play a part in creating novel proteins or medications. It is employed in the study of gene expression, gene sequence analysis, gene molecular modeling, protein 3D structures, the synthesis of bioactive chemicals, and illness detection (30). The software used for drug design purposes is mentioned below.

7.5.1 *Computer-Aided Drug Design*

In finding and developing new drugs, a group of computer-based applications known as computer-aided drug design (CADD) are used to calculate, depict, and manipulate the structures and reactions of molecules. The decrease of time and human resources required for drug discovery is the primary benefit of CADD. Structure-based drug design (SBDD) and ligand-based drug design (LBDD) are the two main categories of CADD techniques (31).

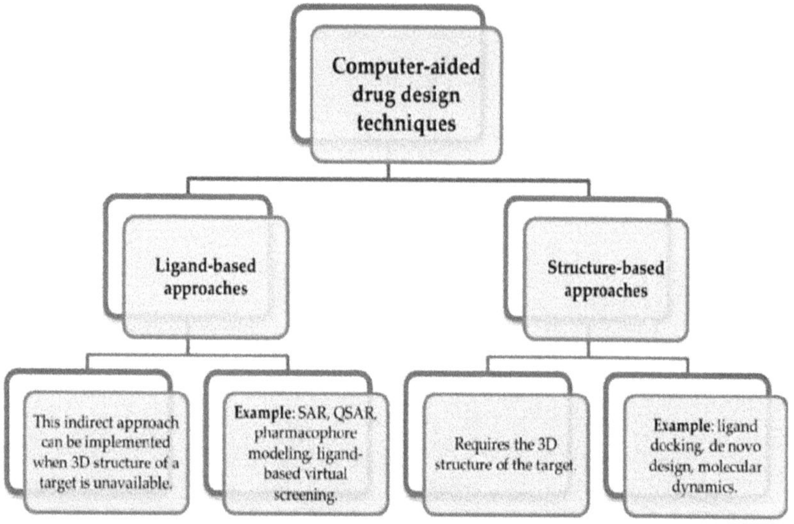

Image 7.6: Types of CADD (32).

CADD is capable of increasing the hit rate of novel drug compounds because it uses a much more targeted search than traditional methods. It not only aims to explain the molecular basis of therapeutic activity but also to predict possible derivatives that would have improved properties (33).

CADD is usually used for three major purposes:

1. Filter large compound libraries into smaller sets of predicted active compounds that can be tested experimentally.

2. Guide the optimization of lead compounds, whether to increase their affinity or optimize drug metabolism and pharmacokinetics (DMPK) properties including absorption, distribution, metabolism, excretion, and the potential for toxicity (ADMET).

3. Design novel compounds, either by "growing" starting molecules one functional group at a time or by piecing together fragments into novel chemotypes (34).

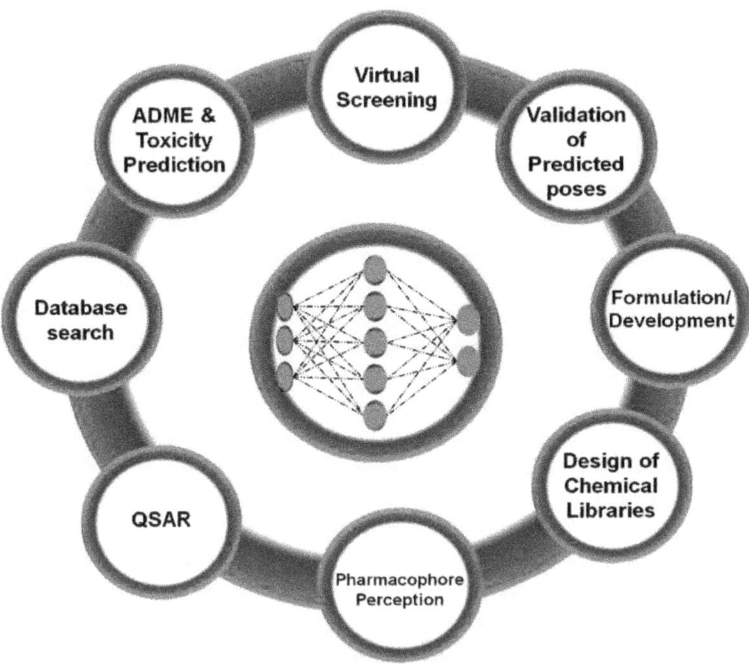

Image 7.7: Drug Design by Using CADD

Examples of CADD software

a) PASS online/ way 2 drug:

The biological activity spectrum of a chemical substance refers to the variety of unique biological activities that result from its interactions with different biological entities (35). It operates under the tenet that a compound's structure and biological activity are equal. The online tool Prediction of Activity Spectra for Substances (PASS) predicts about

4000 distinct types of biological activity, encompassing toxicological, pharmacological, and unpleasant consequences. These encompass impacts on the expression of genes, and interplay with metabolic transporters and enzymes, among other things. The Department of Bioinformatics, Institute of Biomedical Chemistry, Moscow-119121, has used PASS version 2.0 to forecast the activity spectrum of the suggested substance. This version was created in 2011 (36).

Pa (probability "to be active") calculates the likelihood that the substance under study is a member of the class of active compounds (resembles the structures of molecules, which are the most typical in a subset of "actives" in the PASS training set) (37).

Pi (probability "to be inactive") calculates the possibility that the substance under research falls into the category of inactive substances (resembles the structures of molecules. which are the most typical in a sub-set of "inactive" in the PASS training set).

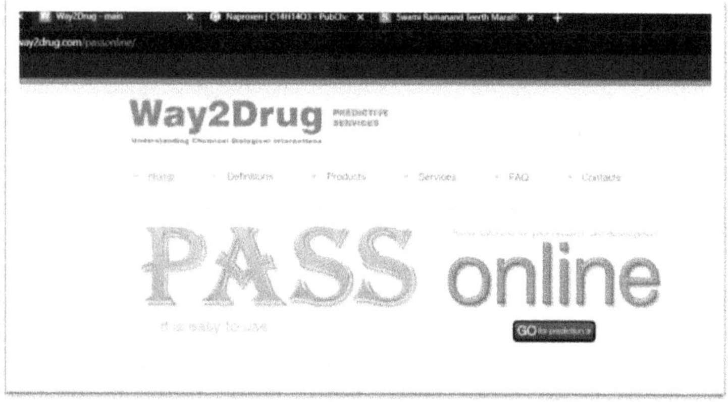

Image 7.8: Interface of PASS online
(http://www.way2drug.Com).

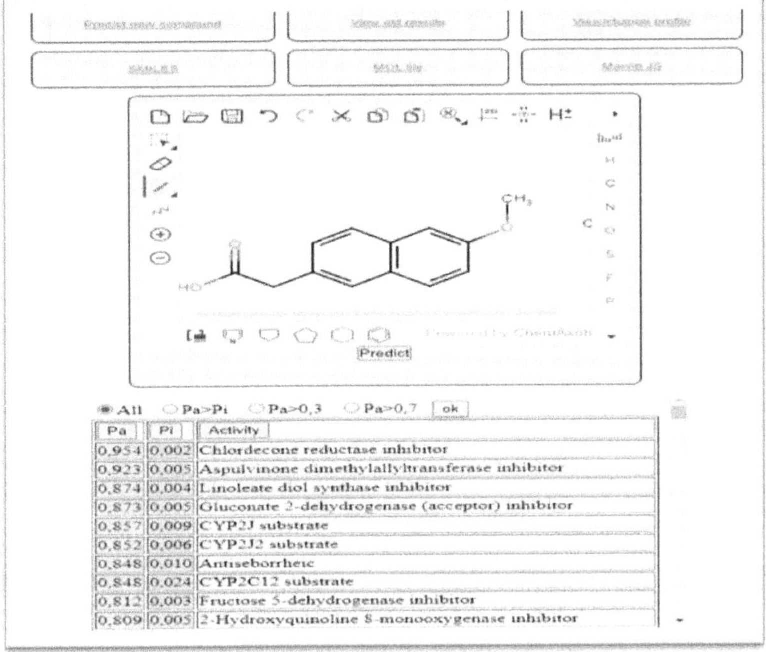

Image 7.9: Result of the PASS Study

b) Molinspiration

The Molinspiration tool offers valuable and precise predictions of various attributes of a ligand by calculating Log P, the number of hydrogen donors and acceptors, the Topological Polar Surface Area (TPSA), and the number of rotatable bonds. This comprehensive analysis aids in assessing the ligand's efficacy and potential biological activity with high reliability and utility. The oral bioavailability of a medicine is determined by its lipophilicity (LogP) and TPSA values. All five ligands' LogP values fell within the range, indicating a high permeability rate for these ligands into cells. due to the lipophilic nature of the phospholipid bilayer (38).

Molinspiration property:

- (TPSA) Topological Polar Surface Area
- mi Log P
- n, Violation
- Rotatable bonds
- Molecular Volume

Bioactivity properties: The bioactivity of the medication can be assessed by computing the activity score of the GPCR ligand, ion channel modulator, nuclear receptor ligand, kinase inhibitor, protease inhibitor, and enzyme inhibitor (39).

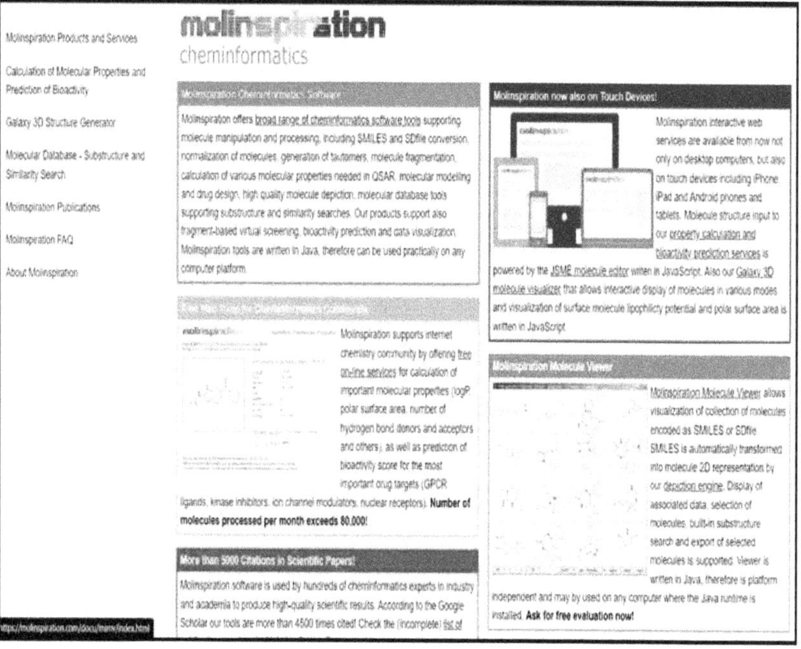

Image 7.10: Interface of molinspiration

(https://molinspiration.com).

c)   Molecular docking

A type of computational modeling known as molecular docking makes it easier to anticipate the preferred binding orientation of one molecule (such as a ligand) to another (such as a receptor) when they combine to form a stable complex. The strength and stability of complexes and their energy profile (such as their binding free energy) can all be predicted using knowledge of the bound molecules' preferred orientation. Utilizing molecular docking, a scoring function is possible (40). Nowadays, molecular docking is frequently used to predict how tiny compounds (potential drugs) will bind to their biomolecular targets (such as proteins, carbohydrates, and nucleic acids) to establish their preliminary binding characteristics. This creates the necessary raw data for the structure-based drug development of new, more specialized, and effective drugs.

The goal of Molecular docking:

Molecular docking aims to achieve an optimized docked conformer of both interacting molecules to reduce the system's free energy. Models for the final anticipated binding free energy (Gbind) include dispersion and repulsion (Gvdw), hydrogen bonds (Ghbond), desolvation (Gdesolv), electrostatic (Gelec), torsional free energy (Gtor), final total internal energy (Gtotal), and the energy of the unbound system (Gunb). As a result, a thorough comprehension of the fundamental ideas that drive predicted binding free energy (Gbind) offers supplementary knowledge about the many types of interactions that motivate molecular docking (41).

Table 7.6: Tools required for Molecular docking.

S. No	Tool Name	About Tool
1.	RCSB PDB Database	RCSB.org is the US data center for the Global Protein Data Bank (PDB), which contains 3D structure data for large biological molecules.
2.	Pub Chem	It is an open chemistry database at the National Institutes of Health (NIH) and a key chemical information resource. **Launched in: 2004**
3.	The Pymol Molecular Graphics System.	Visualizing molecular structures, offering advanced graphics, and rendering capabilities. **Version: 2.3.4** Developed by: Schrodinger LLC
4.	Auto dock Vina (Molecular docking software)	Prediction of ligand-protein interactions and binding affinities. **Version: 1.5.7** Developed by: The Scripps Research Institute.
5.	MGL Tool	Required for file PDBQT file generation **Version: 1.5.7** Developed by: The Scripps Research Institute
6.	Discovery Studio Visualizer (BIOVIA)	Enables comprehensive visualization and analysis of biomolecular structures and properties. **Version: 21.1.0.20298** Developed by: Dassault Systems Biovia Corp.

Over the past 20 years, more than 60 docking tools and programs have been created for academic and commercial use, including DOCK, AutoDock, FlexX, Surflex, and GOLD. Among these programs, AutoDock Vina, GOLD, and MOE-Dock predicted top-ranking poses with the best scores (42).

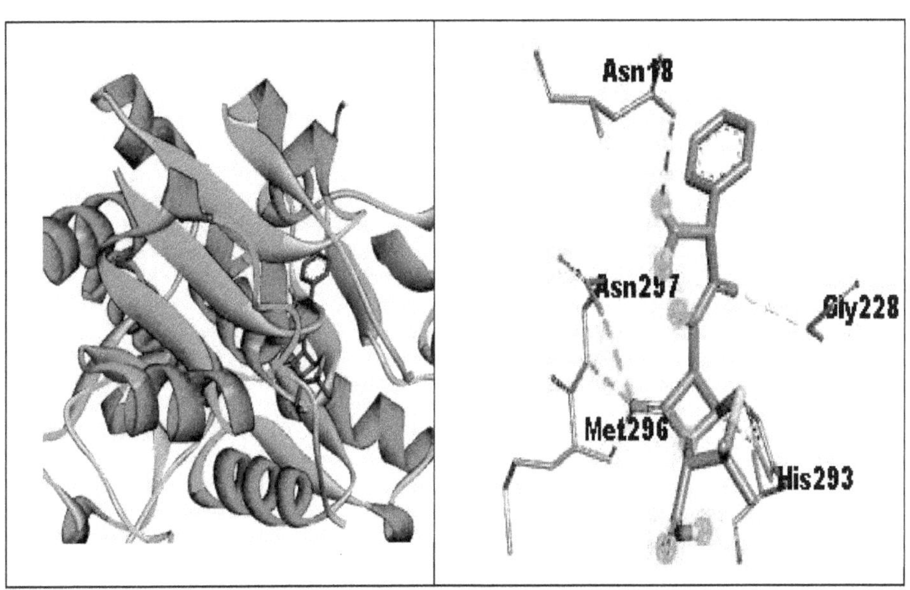

Image 7.11: Receptor & ligand

d) ADMET /Swiss ADME

In pharmacokinetics and pharmacology, the phrase "absorption, distribution, metabolism, and excretion," or ADME, describes how a medication is eliminated from an organism. The four criteria all affect drug levels and the kinetics of drug exposure to tissues, affecting the chemical's performance and pharmacological activity as a medicine. LADME, ADMET, or LADMET are the outcomes when liberation and/or toxicity are considered. In addition to having sufficient activity against the therapeutic target, every researcher should display the appropriate ADMET properties at a therapeutic dose. Consequently, many in silico models are developed to predict the characteristics of the chemical ADMET (43). The tool required for the ADMET Study is-Pre-ADMET, the PREMATABO Family server Designed by Y.M. Kang.

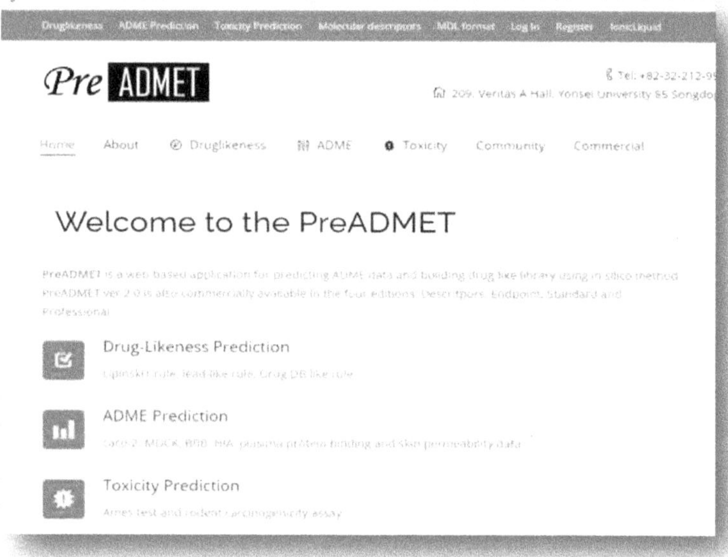

Image 7.12: interface of a pre-ADMET web server (44).

7.5.2   *Molecular Modelling Software*

In chemistry, molecular modeling is an essential technique that helps researchers comprehend and anticipate molecular behavior. It is important because it sheds light on molecules' interactions, structures, and behaviors, which helps with medicine development, materials research, and other scientific pursuits. Molecular modeling is carried out with the aid of multiple software programs.

- ChemDoodle: A user-friendly software for creating chemical 3D structures and managing reaction schemes in real-time.
- Hypercube: Offers functions for protein simulations, molecular modeling, and visualization, with specialized software for protein modeling.
- BIOVIA Draw: Designed for chemists, providing tools for drawing complex molecules, chemical reactions, and biological sequences.

These software tools enable scientists to visualize, analyze, and simulate molecular structures, aiding in research, education, and the advancement of scientific knowledge in chemistry and related fields (45). It helps students visualize and understand chemical concepts, such as electron densities and electrostatic potentials, which are crucial for understanding molecular behavior and reactivity.

- Molecular models can reveal the locations of electrons, chemical bonds, and molecular size, providing insights into molecular structure and bonding (46).
- Used to predict bond lengths, angles, molecular polarity, charge distribution, and quantum mechanical properties such as absorption and emission spectra. However, the computational complexity increases with the number of atoms, making it challenging to model large molecules or systems (15).

Table 7.7: Description of Molecular modeling

Definition	Encompasses all theoretical and computational methods used to model or mimic the behavior of molecules.
Applications	Used in computational chemistry, drug design, computational biology, and materials science.
Scope	Studies molecular systems ranging from small chemical systems to large biological molecules and material assemblies.
Techniques	It includes molecular mechanics and quantum chemistry approaches for an atomistic-level description of molecular systems.
Molecular Mechanics	Uses classical mechanics to describe the physical basis behind models, where atoms are seen as point charges with associated

7.6 Key AI tools for PhD programs

7.6.1 *ChatGPT*

ChatGPT stands for "Chat Generative Pre-Trained Transformer." It's a variant of the GPT model developed by OpenAI. It is a powerful tool that can be utilized in various stages of PhD thesis writing and article publication, as well as overcoming writer's block. It provides help in the following ways:

- Research Assistance
- Writing Support
- Feedback and Revision
- Exploratory Analysis
- Data Interpretation
- Problem Solving

- Collaboration Facilitation
- 24/7 Availability (47).

7.6.2   *Gamma*

Gamma AI is a presentation tool that revolutionizes how ideas are delivered using artificial intelligence. It enables users to quickly and easily produce captivating material, such as papers, presentations, and webpages, with little need for design or formatting.

Key features of Gamma AI include:

- AI-Powered Content Generation
- Live Presentation Mode
- Embedding Capabilities
- Built-in Analytics
- Collaborative Features
- Cross-Device Compatibility (48).

Gamma AI's AI-powered system assists users in creating beautiful and engaging content, providing a more streamlined and efficient way to create presentations compared to traditional tools like PowerPoint and Google Slides (49).

7.6.3   *Slides.AI*

Another presentation tool that makes remote team collaboration easier is Slide.AI, which lets users assign assignments, track presentations, and receive feedback all from within their workspace. The following characteristics of the tool improve the process of creating presentations

- AI Native

- Modern Decks
- Frictionless Design
- Collaboration
- Built-in Style and Layout Variations.

Slide.AI is a powerful tool for creating engaging and interactive presentations with minimal design and formatting work required, making it ideal for a wide range of use cases, including business presentations, educational lectures, webpage design, collaborative projects, and interactive content sharing (50).

7.6.4   *Perplexity*

Perplexity AI is a tool that offers various advantages for users, especially in the context of PhD thesis writing. Perplexity AI can benefit thesis writing based on the provided sources or references.

- Accurate Information: Guarantees factual accuracy in content provider, offering current and accurate data for thesis research.
- Versatility: This adaptable tool is ideal for researchers, students, and content creators; individuals pursuing advanced education and engaging in comprehensive projects will find it helpful.
- Customizing Research: With Perplexity AI's features like Focus, Co-pilot, and Vision, users may customize searches, concentrate on specific terms, and even upload images for analysis(51).

It aids researchers in analyzing and improving their thesis's linguistic coherence, clarity, and flow. By providing insights into language complexity and coherence, Perplexity.ai helps researchers refine their arguments and ensure the comprehensibility of their work, ultimately enhancing the overall quality and impact of the thesis (52).

7.6.5   *Write Sonic*

Write Sonic.ai provides advanced text creation and editing features. Its features—which help scholars improve the overall coherence and clarity of their theses—include language refinement, style adjustment, and content expansion. It can help organize and explain complex concepts by combining other languages and suggesting structural modifications. With the help of these tools, researchers can write PhD theses more quickly and effectively while also improving the caliber of their work (53).

Other AI tools in writing

- WordAI
- Copy.ai
- SEO.ai
- Wordtune
- Simplified
- DeepL
- Hypotenuse AI
- Etc.

7.7 References

1.   Priya Pedamkar. Types of Computer Software. 2023.

2. Ngulube P. Improving the quality of reporting findings using computer data analysis applications in educational research in context. Heliyon. 2023 Sep;9(9): e19683.

3. What is citation management software? Research guide. 2024.

4. Deacon A, Jaftha J, Horwitz D. Customising Microsoft Office to develop a tutorial learning environment. Brit J Educational Tech. 2004 Mar;35(2):223–34.

5. Divisi D, Di Leonardo G, Zaccagna G, Crisci R. Basic statistics with Microsoft Excel: a review. J Thorac Dis. 2017 Jun;9(6):1734–40.

6. Hashemi M, Azizinezhad M, Farokhi M. Power Point as an innovative tool for teaching and learning in modern classes. Procedia - Social and Behavioral Sciences. 2012; 31:559–63.

7. Li Z, Wan H, Shi Y, Ouyang P. Personal Experience with Four Kinds of Chemical Structure Drawing Software: Review on ChemDraw, ChemWindow, ISIS/Draw, and ChemSketch. J Chem Inf Comput Sci. 2004 Sep 1;44(5):1886–90.

8. Raiyn J, Rayan A. How Chemicals' Drawing and Modeling Improve Chemistry Teaching in Colleges of Education. World Journal of Chemical Education.

9. Peterson JJ, Snee RD, McAllister PR, Schofield TL, Carella AJ. Statistics in Pharmaceutical Development and Manufacturing. Journal of Quality Technology. 2009 Apr;41(2):111–34.

10. Fitria TN. QuillBot as an online tool: Students' alternative in paraphrasing and rewriting of English writing. EJ. 2021 Nov 7;9(1):183.

11. Chikkam, Shanmuka Gopala Krishna. Plagiarism Checker. 2023;

12. Orlando J, Hanham J, Ullman J. Exploring intentional use of a technological proxy, Turnitin, to enhance student academic literacy practices. AJET [Internet]. 2018 Sep 16 [cited 2024 Apr 11];34(4). Available from: https://ajet.org.au/index.php/AJET/article/view/3575

13. Fitria TN. Grammarly as AI-powered English Writing Assistant: Students' Alternative for Writing English. MetathesisJEnglLangLitTeach. 2021 May 18;5(1):65.

14. Nguyen DG, Funk J, Robbins JB, Crogan-Grundy C, Presnell SC, Singer T, et al. Bioprinted 3D Primary Liver Tissues Allow Assessment of Organ-Level Response to Clinical Drug-Induced Toxicity In Vitro. Van Grunsven LA, editor. PLoS ONE. 2016 Jul 7;11(7):e0158674.

15. Voet A, Qing X, Lee XY, De Raeymaecker J, Tame J, Zhang K, et al. Pharmacophore modeling: advances, limitations, and current utility in drug discovery. JRLCR. 2014 Nov;81.

16. Campbell Robertson. Nielsen Brings a New Marketing Strategy to Broadway. 2020;

17. Microsoft Excel analyzes data [Internet]. Available from: https://softwarekeep.com/blogs/tips-and-tricks/excel-data-analysis-tools

18. Cooksey RW. Descriptive Statistics for Summarising Data. In: Illustrating Statistical Procedures: Finding Meaning in Quantitative Data [Internet]. Singapore: Springer Singapore; 2020 [cited 2024 Apr 11]. p. 61–139. Available from: http://link.springer.com/10.1007/978-981-15-2537-7_5

19. Rodriguez RN. SAS. WIREs Computational Stats. 2011 Jan;3(1):1–11.

20. Freund, Rudolf, and Ramon Littell. SAS system for regression. John Wiley & Sons; 2000.

21. Dmitrienko, Alex, Christy Chuang-Stein, and Ralph B. D'Agostino Sr. Pharmaceutical statistics using SAS: a practical guide. SAS Institute. 2007;

22. Das Sarkar R. Pharma Software - A Complete Overview. Int J Sci Healthcare Res. 2023 Apr 28;8(2):166–77.

23. Diaby V, Adunlin G, Montero AJ. Survival Modeling for the Estimation of Transition Probabilities in Model-Based Economic Evaluations in the Absence of Individual Patient Data: A Tutorial. PharmacoEconomics. 2014 Feb;32(2):101–8.

24. Spurling GK, Mansfield PR, Montgomery BD, Lexchin J, Doust J, Othman N, et al. Information from Pharmaceutical Companies and the Quality, Quantity, and Cost of Physicians' Prescribing: A Systematic Review. Henry D, editor. PLoS Med. 2010 Oct 19;7(10): e1000352.

25. Lo, Yu-Chen, Ren Gui, Hiroshi Honda, and Jorge Z. Torres. Quantitative Methods in System-Based Drug Discovery.". In: In CSystems, Sustainability and Innovation. IntechOpen; 2016.

26. Motulsky, H. J. Prism 5 statistics guide. 2007;31(1):39–42.

27. Chertin B, Pollack A, Koulikov D, Rabinowitz R, Hain D, Hadas-Halpren I, et al. Conservative Treatment of Ureteropelvic Junction Obstruction in Children with Antenatal Diagnosis of Hydronephrosis: Lessons Learned after 16 Years of Follow-Up. European Urology. 2006 Apr;49(4):734–9.

28. Berkman SJ, Roscoe EM, Bourret JC. Comparing self-directed methods for training staff to create graphs using GraphPad Prism. J of App Behav Analysis. 2019 Feb;52(1):188–204.

29. De García SO, García-Encina PA, Irusta-Mata R. Dose-response behavior of the bacterium Vibrio fischeri exposed to pharmaceuticals and personal care products. Ecotoxicology. 2016 Jan;25(1):141–62.

30. Pal R, Pandey P, Thakur SK, Chanana A, Singh RP. Drug Design and Development Involving Novel Software In Pharmaceuticals. 2022;

31. Osakwe, Odilia, and S. A. A. Rizv. The significance of discovery screening and structure optimization studies." Social aspects of drug discovery, development, and commercialization. In 2016. p. 109–28.

32. Prasad S, Srivastava A, Singh N, Singh H, Saluja R, Kumar A, et al. Present and future challenges in therapeutic designing using computational approaches. In: Computational Approaches for Novel Therapeutic and Diagnostic Designing to Mitigate SARS-CoV-2 Infection [Internet]. Elsevier; 2022 [cited 2024 Apr 11]. p. 489–505. Available from: https://linkinghub.elsevier.com/retrieve/pii/B9780323911726000200

33. Lin X, Li X, Lin X. A Review on Applications of Computational Methods in Drug Screening and Design. Molecules. 2020 Mar 18;25(6):1375.

34. Zhao L, Ciallella HL, Aleksunes LM, Zhu H. Advancing computer-aided drug discovery (CADD) by big data and data-driven machine learning modeling. Drug Discovery Today. 2020 Sep;25(9):1624–38.

35. Fliri AF, Loging WT, Thadeio PF, Volkmann RA. Biological spectra analysis: Linking biological activity profiles to molecular structure. Proc Natl Acad Sci USA. 2005 Jan 11;102(2):261–6.

36. Stepanchikova A, Lagunin A, Filimonov D, Poroikov V. Prediction of Biological Activity Spectra for Substances: Evaluation on the Diverse Sets of Drug-Like Structures. CMC. 2003 Feb 1;10(3):225–33.

37. Filimonov DA, Lagunin AA, Gloriozova TA, Rudik AV, Druzhilovskii DS, Pogodin PV, et al. Prediction of the Biological Activity Spectra of Organic Compounds Using the Pass Online Web Resource. Chem Heterocycl Comp. 2014 Jun;50(3):444–57.

38. Kuchana, Madhavi, Maneesha Pulavarthi, Sasikala Potthuri, Vyshnavi Manduri, and Vijaya Durga Jaggarapu. In silico study of molecular properties, bioactivity, and toxicity of 2- (substituted benzylidene) succinic acids and some selected anti-inflammatory drugs. Int J Pharm Sci Drug Res. 2020;12(4):353–9.

39. Husain A, Ahmad A, Khan SA, Asif M, Bhutani R, Al-Abbasi FA. Synthesis, molecular properties, toxicity, and biological evaluation of some new substituted imidazolidine derivatives in search of potent anti-inflammatory agents. Saudi Pharmaceutical Journal. 2016 Jan;24(1):104–14.

40. Novikov FN, Chilov GG. Molecular docking: theoretical background, practical applications, and perspectives. Mendeleev Communications. 2009 Sep;19(5):237–42.

41. Pagadala NS, Syed K, Tuszynski J. Software for molecular docking: a review. Biophys Rev. 2017 Apr;9(2):91–102.

42. Lamb ML, Jorgensen WL. Computational approaches to molecular recognition. Current Opinion in Chemical Biology. 1997 Dec;1(4):449–57.

43. Kar S, Leszczynski J. Open access in silico tools to predict the ADMET profiling of drug candidates. Expert Opinion on Drug Discovery. 2020 Dec 1;15(12):1473–87.

44. Moroy G, Martiny VY, Vayer P, Villoutreix BO, Miteva MA. Toward in silico structure-based ADMET prediction in drug discovery. Drug Discovery Today. 2012 Jan;17(1–2):44–55.

45. Yang SY. Pharmacophore modeling and applications in drug discovery: challenges and recent advances. Drug Discovery Today. 2010 Jun;15(11–12):444–50.

46. McGregor MJ, Muskal SM. Pharmacophore Fingerprinting. 1. Application to QSAR and Focused Library Design. J Chem Inf Comput Sci. 1999 May 25;39(3):569–74.

47. Sallam M. The Utility of ChatGPT as an Example of Large Language Models in Healthcare Education, Research and Practice: Systematic Review on the Future Perspectives and Potential Limitations [Internet]. 2023 [cited 2024 Apr 12]. Available from: http://medrxiv.org/lookup/doi/10.1101/2023.02.19.23286155

48. Shamsuddinova S, Heryani P, Naval MA. Evolution to revolution: Critical exploration of educators' perceptions of the impact of Artificial Intelligence (AI) on the teaching and learning process in the GCC region. International Journal of Educational Research. 2024; 125:102326.

49. Ruksana, T.P. Unveiling ChatGPT's Influence in Education. Journal of Applied Science, Engineering, Technology and Management. 2024;2(1):9–14.

50. Zheng C, Wang D, Wang AY, Ma X. Telling Stories from Computational Notebooks: AI-Assisted Presentation Slides Creation for Presenting Data Science Work. In: CHI Conference on Human Factors in Computing Systems [Internet]. New Orleans LA USA: ACM; 2022 [cited 2024 Apr 12]. p. 1–20. Available from: https://dl.acm.org/doi/10.1145/3491102.3517615

51. Khan R, Gupta N, Sinhababu A, Chakravarty R. Impact of Conversational and Generative AI Systems on Libraries: A Use Case Large Language Model (LLM). Science & Technology Libraries. 2023 Sep 11;1–15.

52. Lily, Jaratin, Mori Kogid, Debbra Toria Nipo, Abd Karim, and Mohd Rahimie. AI Tools For Postgraduate Academic Research (Part 2): Exploring Innovative AI Tools For Idea Generation. 2023.

53. Lukac D, Lazareva A. Artificial Intelligence and Educational Assessment System Landscape, Challenges And Ways To Tackle AI-based Plagiarism. In Palma, Spain; 2023 [Cited 2024 Apr 12]. P. 953–62. Available From: Https://Library.iated.org/view/LUKAC2023ART.

Chapter 8

THESIS DEFENCE

Defended thesis, affirmed contribution.

8.1 Overview

The thesis defence is sometimes called an oral or viva voce defence. A research scholar delivers and defends their thesis or dissertation in front of a committee of subject-matter experts as part of the final examination for a research degree. The study findings are usually presented, and then the committee members assess the student's knowledge, comprehension, and contribution to the subject during a Q&A session. Passing the thesis defence is an essential step to obtain a research degree. Before the thesis defence, it is important to remember these important points.

8.2 Grasp the significant findings and objectives outlined in the thesis

a) **Clarity of objectives:** Preparing to present your thesis requires a comprehensive understanding of primary findings and objectives. Thus, at the time of presentation, readers should understand what specific questions or problems the thesis aims to address.

b) **Significance of findings**: Understand why the thesis's major findings matter. How do they contribute to existing knowledge in the field? What implications do they have for theory, practice, or further research?

c) **Contextualization:** Provide context for the major findings by discussing the background literature and research that informed the thesis. This helps readers understand how the findings fit into the broader scholarly conversation (1).

d) **Highlighting key contributions:** Identify the thesis's unique contributions. What new insights, methods, or perspectives does it offer? Emphasize the originality and significance of these contributions (2).

e) **Summarization:** Summarize the major findings and objectives concisely. This helps readers grasp the essence of the thesis and prepares them for a more detailed discussion during the defense.

8.3 Crafting of Effective Presentation

Telling a gripping tale about your research journey is similar to creating a strong presentation for your thesis defense.

a) **Clear structure:** Start with a clear outline that guides your audience through your presentation. Introduce your topic, state your objectives, present your findings, and conclude with key takeaways.

b) **Appealing introduction:** Begin with a hook to grab your audience's attention. Explain why your research is essential and how it contributes to the field.

c) **Visual appeal:** Use visually appealing slides that are easy to read. Incorporate images, graphs, and charts to illustrate key points. Visual representations can enhance understanding and retention for both the author and the audience (3).

d) **Simple language:** Explain your ideas using simple, straightforward language. Imagine you are explaining your research to someone who knows nothing about your field.

e) **Tell a story:** Frame your presentation as a story with a beginning, middle, and end. Take your audience through your research process, highlighting challenges, discoveries, and insights.

f)   **Engage the audience:** Keep your audience engaged by asking questions, encouraging participation, make them feel like active participants in your presentation, not passive observers.

g)   **Stay organized:** Keep your presentation organized and focused. Stick to your allotted time and avoid going off on tangents. If you have too much information, prioritize the most important points and save the rest (4).

8.4 Practice for the presentation

Practicing your presentation will ensure that everything goes smoothly and confidently like fine-tuning an instrument before a concert. Practice your speech several times, paying attention to the material and delivery. To identify any anxious tendencies or places that need work, practice in front of a mirror or record yourself. Consider asking for helpful criticism from friends, family, or coworkers after presenting. Embrace any nerves as natural, and use practice sessions to build confidence in your material. The more you practice, the more comfortable and polished your presentation will become, setting you up for success on the big day. Show confidence in your research by speaking clearly and passionately. Believe in the value of your work and let your enthusiasm shine through. Your passion will inspire others to care about your research too (5,6).

8.5 Anticipate potential questions

To properly defend your thesis, you must prepare comprehensive responses to any queries you may have. It entails thinking through any questions your audience could have regarding your study and being ready to respond concisely and comprehensively. Review your thesis in detail and mark any points that need clarification or may lead to further questioning. Think about the importance of your study, the approach you took, and the conclusions you came to. After you've determined what questions to ask, give careful attention to your answers. To ensure you can speak clearly and confidently when responding to these questions during the presentation, practice your responses.

Being well-prepared to address potential questions demonstrates your expertise and strengthens your overall presentation. Do not be afraid to admit that if you do not know the answer, you should use it as an opportunity to engage in a constructive discussion (7,8). We have enlisted specific criteria for potential questions that can be asked during the thesis defence.

a) Clarification/ methodological questions:

- Can you clarify your methodology/approach?
- Can you clarify the terminology used in your thesis?
- How did you select your sample population?
- What specific techniques or tools did you use to collect data?
- Could you provide more detail on how you analyzed your data?
- How did you ensure the validity and reliability of your findings?
- Can you clarify any ambiguous or unclear points in your thesis?
- What considerations did you take into account when designing your research instruments?
- Could you explain any deviations from your initial research plan and the reasons behind them?
- Can you discuss the strengths and limitations of your chosen research methodology?

b) Theoretical questions:

- How does your research contribute to the theoretical understanding of the specific topic?
- Can you explain the theoretical framework that guided your research?
- What theories or models from the literature did you draw upon to develop your hypotheses?
- How do your findings align with or challenge existing theoretical perspectives in the field?
- Can you discuss any theoretical implications of your findings?
- Did you encounter any discrepancies between your theoretical framework and your empirical results? If so, how did you address them?
- How might your research expand or refine existing theories in the field?
- What theoretical perspectives did you consider when interpreting your results?
- Can you articulate the broader theoretical significance of your research within the context of the discipline?
- How does your research contribute to advancing theoretical debates or addressing gaps in the literature?

c) **Significance questions:**
- Why is your research important?
- What motivated you to undertake this research?
- Can you explain the practical significance of your findings?
- How does your research address a gap or issue in the existing literature?

- What are the potential implications of your research for practitioners or policymakers?
- Can you discuss any societal or real-world relevance of your research findings?
- Can you articulate the potential long-term impact of your research?
- What value does your research add to the academic community or society as a whole?

d) Limitation questions:

- What are the main limitations of your study?
- Can you discuss any potential biases in your research design or methodology?
- How might the limitations of your study affect the interpretation of your findings?
- Were there any constraints or challenges that influenced the scope of your research?
- Can you explain how you addressed or mitigated potential limitations in your study?
- What alternative approaches or methodologies could have addressed the limitations of your study?

e) Interpretation questions:

- How do you interpret the key findings of your study?
- Can you explain the significance of [specific result] in the context of your research?
- What factors might influence the interpretation of your research findings?

- How do your findings align with or diverge from previous research in the field?
- Can you discuss any unexpected or contradictory results and their potential implications?
- How might different theoretical perspectives influence the interpretation of your findings?

f) Future directions questions:

- What are the potential avenues for further research based on your findings?
- Can you identify any unanswered questions or gaps in the literature that your research opens up?
- How might your study lay the groundwork for future investigations in the field?
- Are there specific areas or topics that emerged from your research that warrant further exploration?
- Can you discuss potential extensions or refinements of your research methodology for future studies?
- How might advancements in technology or changes in the field influence future research directions?
- Can you propose potential research questions or hypotheses that could build upon the findings of your study?
- Are there interdisciplinary connections or collaborations that could enhance future research in this area?
- Can you outline a potential research agenda based on the implications of your findings?
- How can your research findings be applied in real-world scenarios?

- How do you envision your research contributing to advancing knowledge and addressing challenges in the field in the long term?

You will feel secure and prepared to answer queries during your thesis defense if you anticipate them and have prepared answers.

8.6 Several tricks to captivate your presentation

- Start strong with something interesting to grab attention, like a remarkable fact or a powerful quote.

- Use visuals like slides or graphs to show your main points clearly.

- Tell your presentation like a story, taking your audience through your research journey step by step.

- Get your audience involved by asking questions and inviting them to share their thoughts.

- Keep it short and focused on the essential parts of your research.

- Change up how you speak and move to keep people interested.

- Practice a lot to feel confident and professional when you present.

- Finish with a bang by summarizing your main ideas and leaving your audience with a question to think about or something they can do based on your research (9,10).

8.7 References

1. Cheung YL. Understanding the Writing of Thesis Introductions: An Exploratory Study. Procedia - Social and Behavioral Sciences. 2012; 46:744–9.
2. Muhammad Shaheen. The Concept of Originality in Academic Research of Engineering. 2021.
3. Pokharel, S.D. Some Suggestions to Defend Viva-voce Successfully. PRAGYAN A Peer Reviewed Multidisciplinary Journal. 2021;3(1):188–95.
4. Bitzer, E. M., Vernon Trafford, and Shosh Leshem. The doctoral viva voce is a rite of passage into academia. 2018.
5. Pahls, Rev Michael JG. Dissertation Defense Presentation. 2015.
6. Ekong, A.O. and Udukeke, F.O. Oral Presentations In Educational Research: An Example. In Education. 131.
7. Lantsoght EOL. Effectiveness of Doctoral Defense Preparation Methods. Education Sciences. 2022 Jul 8;12(7):473.
8. Murray, Rowena. How to Survive Your Viva: Defending a Thesis in an Oral Examination. [United Kingdom]: McGraw-Hill Education; 2015.
9. Lantsoght EOL. Preparation for the Doctoral Defense: Methods and Relation to Defense Outcome and Perception [Internet]. 2021 [cited 2024 Apr 12]. Available from: https://www.preprints.org/manuscript/202109.0481/v1
10. Roberts CM. The dissertation journey: a practical and comprehensive guide to planning, writing, and defending your dissertation. 2nd ed. Thousand Oaks, Calif: Corwin Press; 2010. 229 p.

Chapter 9

EFFECTIVE FINDINGS DISSEMINATION

Translating findings into actionable knowledge.

9.1 Overview

In the ever-changing world of higher education, research, and innovation, making a discovery is just half the story. Any discovery's real potential can be realized through its dissemination—the skill of imparting knowledge to a global audience. Good research findings are disseminated to policymakers, practitioners, and the public beyond academic publications and lab walls. It is the cornerstone of progress, igniting societal advancement and turning ideas into action. It serves as a catalyst for change, encouraging creativity, guiding judgment, and influencing the public's perception of urgent problems (1). By facilitating the exchange of ideas and evidence-based practices, dissemination bridges the gap between theory and practice, academia and industry, research, and policy. We can disseminate our ideas or innovations in several ways:

- Publication in academic journals.
- Presentation at conferences and seminars.
- Sharing on online platforms and repositories.
- Collaboration with media for press coverage.
- Engagement with communities and stakeholders.
- Crafting policy briefs for policymakers.
- Organizing workshops and training sessions.
- Utilizing social media and blogging.
- Forming collaborative partnerships with industry.
- Developing educational materials for broader audiences (2). In the subsequent section, we will delve into the significance of academic journal publication within the PhD program and highlight its pivotal role in scholarly advancement.

9.2 Publication in academic journals

Publication in academic publications is essential to provide a comprehensive picture of scholarly research. This is especially true for PhD programs. The following actions are involved:

9.2.1   Prepare the manuscript

Clear and logical organization of your research findings is necessary while preparing a manuscript. Begin by organizing the document and defining its key themes. Utilize headers and subheadings to help your reader navigate your writing and write in clear, succinct language. Make careful to style your manuscript correctly and give due credit to all sources. To ensure your paper is error-free, proofread it thoroughly for grammatical, spelling, and formatting mistakes before submitting it. It's vital to remember that each journal has different policies and procedures when you prepare to submit your work for publication. While these guidelines may vary slightly, most journals follow a similar structure for manuscripts. An abstract will normally come first, followed by the introduction, composed of three key sections: background, your creative research, and your primary conclusions. The material and methods part must then be covered, and then the results, discussion, conclusion, and references (3,4).

Researchers should follow these guidelines when writing their manuscripts. They should also keep their original draft handy to easily tweak it to fit different journal requirements. This approach can save them time and effort, smoothing the publication process.

9.2.2   *Identifying suitable journals for publication*

Selecting the ideal journal for publication doesn't have to be difficult. By reviewing the objectives and coverage of the publication, any researcher can quickly identify the ideal fit. The journal's homepage often has this information available. It is considerably simpler if a student is working on a project related to a certain subject, such as pharmaceutics, pharmacognosy, or pharmacology. Simply seek out journals that are focused on those domains. For example, students must locate a pharmaceutics publication if the study subject concerns medication compositions. By following these strategies, any researcher can quickly identify the ideal journal for their work. It's all about matching research projects with the right audience and domain expertise (5). We have also suggested some strategies/ criteria for finding suitable journals for your research findings.

- **Scope match:** Ensure the journal's scope corresponds with your research. Check previous issues to see whether they have published anything on related subjects.

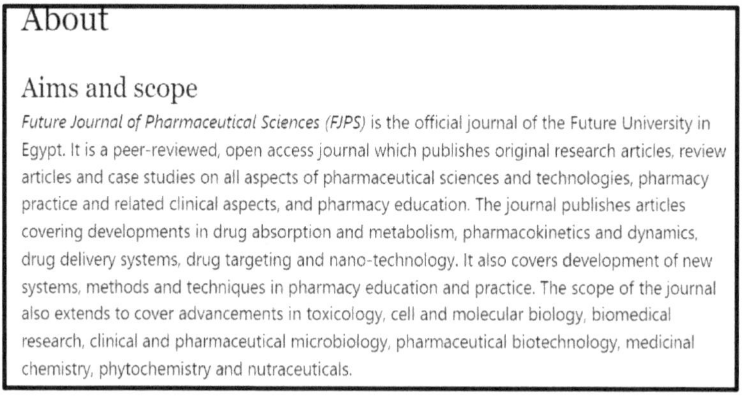

About

Aims and scope

Future Journal of Pharmaceutical Sciences (FJPS) is the official journal of the Future University in Egypt. It is a peer-reviewed, open access journal which publishes original research articles, review articles and case studies on all aspects of pharmaceutical sciences and technologies, pharmacy practice and related clinical aspects, and pharmacy education. The journal publishes articles covering developments in drug absorption and metabolism, pharmacokinetics and dynamics, drug delivery systems, drug targeting and nano-technology. It also covers development of new systems, methods and techniques in pharmacy education and practice. The scope of the journal also extends to cover advancements in toxicology, cell and molecular biology, biomedical research, clinical and pharmaceutical microbiology, pharmaceutical biotechnology, medicinal chemistry, phytochemistry and nutraceuticals.

Image 9.1: Screenshot of the aim and scope of the journal.

- **Audience fit:** Consider the journal's audience. Will your findings be relevant and interesting to them?

- **Impact factor:** Check the journal's impact factor to gauge its influence in the field. Higher impact factors often indicate more prestigious journals. Often, it requires more novel and high-quality data (6).

- **Peer review process**: Examine the journal's peer review procedure. Is it strict? Peer review protects the standards and integrity of scholarly publications, ensuring that the academic community only receives rigorous and reliable research.

- **Publication frequency**: Consider how often the journal publishes. Will your research fit their schedule? Generally, a monthly journal can give you a quick response, saving you time.

- **Open access options**: Open access options refer to publishing models that make research articles freely available to readers without requiring a subscription or payment. This can increase the visibility and accessibility of your work. Alternative publishing models are available beyond open access, including traditional subscription-based models like hybrid and gold open access.

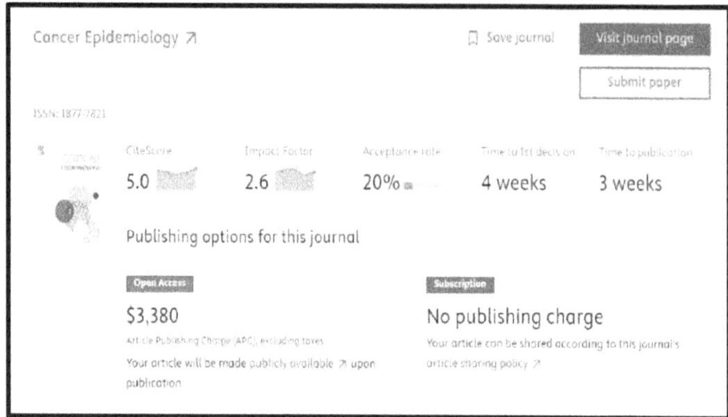

Image 9.2: Screenshot of publishing model along with impact factor and acceptance rate.

- **Reputation:** Verify the journal's and its publisher's reputations. reputable journals maintain the integrity and standards of academia. For instance, Web of Science, indexed by Scopus, UGC, etc. Researchers can use the journal search feature on the Scopus website to find out if a journal is indexed in the database (7). To determine if a journal is indexed in the Web of Science, researchers can access the Web of Science database or the Master Journal List available on the Clarivate Analytics website (8).

- **Acceptance rate:** The term "acceptance rate" describes the proportion of submitted papers approved for publication by a journal following the peer review process. This statistic influences authors' opinions and the academic community's evaluation of the journal's effect and prestige. It measures the selectivity and editorial standards of a journal. For example, a very low acceptance rate indicates that there have been few opportunities for paper acceptance, which can occasionally waste our time and effort. Therefore, it is essential to verify the acceptance rate in addition to the other items.

- **Journal finder:** A journal finder is a platform or service that helps researchers find journals appropriate for their manuscript submissions based on various criteria, including subject area, scope, impact factor, abstract, keywords, title, and acceptance rate. By streamlining the journal selection process, these tools improve authors' chances of successful publication by assisting them in identifying suitable publication sites. Examples include Wiley, Taylor & Francis, Elsevier Journal Finder, etc.

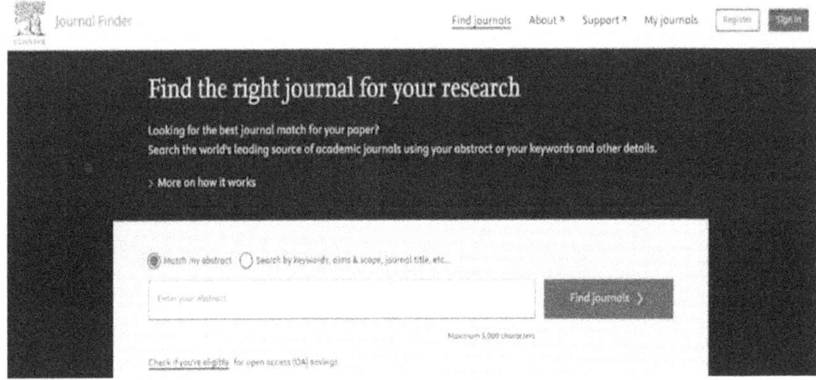

Image 9.3: Screenshot of Elsevier's journal finder tool page

By considering these factors, you can identify journals that best fit your research and increase your chances of successful publication.

9.2.3   Convert manuscript as per journal guidelines

- **Review guidelines**: Carefully read the journal's guidelines authors provided on their website. Adjust the manuscript to match the journal's formatting requirements for fonts, margins, spacing, etc.

- **Sections:** Make sure the manuscript has all the necessary sections—abstract, introduction, methodology, results, discussion, and references—in the sequence that the journal specifies. Verify that writing follows the language, tone, and style preferences specified in the journal.

- **Citations and references:** Format citations and references according to the journal's preferred style guide (e.g., APA, MLA, Chicago). Format figures and tables to meet the journal's specifications regarding size, resolution, and placement within the text.

- **Cover letter:** Write a cover letter that addresses any specific requirements mentioned in the guidelines and highlights why your research is a good fit for the journal.

By following these steps, the Manuscript meets the journal's guidelines and increases the chances of acceptance for publication (9).

9.2.4   Registration and submit

Every researcher or author must follow the following steps to submit research work as a manuscript.

- **Create an account**: Go to the journal's website and create an account. This allows the author to track submissions and receive updates.

Check submission requirements: Review the journal's guidelines to ensure the manuscript meets all the criteria.

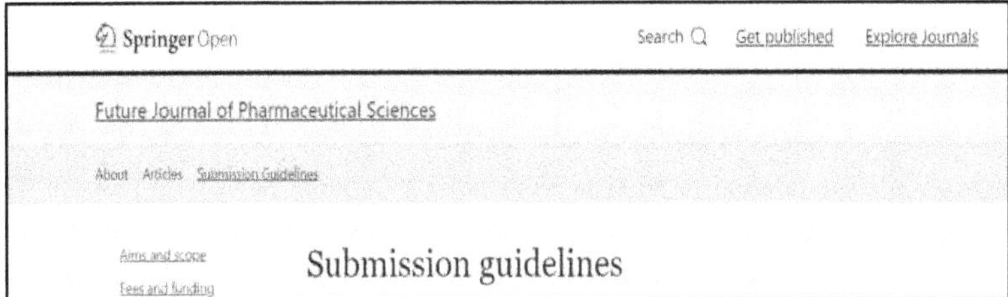

Image 9.4: Screenshot of submission guidelines section.

- **Prepare the manuscript**: Format the manuscript according to the journal's guidelines, including any specific formatting for figures, tables, and references. etc

- **Upload files:** Upload all necessary files to the "upload" section. Journals typically require the main manuscript document (in Word or PDF format), figures, tables, supplementary materials (if any), and any additional files (cover letter, copyright, etc.) requested by the journal.

- **Submit online**: Use the journal's online submission system. Once satisfied with your submission, click the "Submit" or "Finish Submission" button to complete the process.

- **Track progress**: Monitor the submission status through the journal's submission system. The author may receive notifications about the review process or requests for revisions.

- **Respond to reviews:** If the manuscript undergoes peer review, promptly address any reviewer feedback or suggestions.

- **Follow-up:** If the author has not heard back within the expected

- timeframe, do not hesitate to follow up with the journal's editorial office for updates on the status of the submission (10,11).

9.2.5   *Responding to reviewer feedback*

Review all of the reviewers' comments on the submitted manuscript carefully.

- **Take notes:** Take notes on the specific comments and suggestions made by the reviewers for each section of the manuscript. Address each point raised by the reviewers in your response letter, providing clear explanations or revisions where necessary.

- **Be gracious:** Thank the reviewers for their time and valuable feedback, even if some comments may be critical. Constructively respond to critiques, politely explaining disagreements and providing a rationale for your decisions.

- **Make revisions**: Edit your text with the suggestions you've received to make it more accurate, relevant, and clear. To make it simpler for the editors and reviewers to keep track of your modifications, indicate or underline the changes you have made in your revised manuscript.

- **Meet deadlines**: Ensure you meet any deadlines for submitting your revised manuscript and response letter. If there are any unclear or conflicting comments from the reviewers, do not hesitate to seek clarification from the journal's editorial team. Stay positive and resilient throughout the process, understanding that reviewer feedback is an opportunity for improvement and strengthening your research. can adeptly address reviewer feedback, thereby enhancing the (12,13).

9.3 References

1. Ashcraft LE, Quinn DA, Brownson RC. Strategies for effective dissemination of research to United States policymakers: a systematic review. Implementation Sci. 2020 Dec;15(1):89.
2. Ross-Hellauer T, Tennant JP, Banelytė V, Gorogh E, Luzi D, Kraker P, et al. Ten simple rules for innovative dissemination of research. Schwartz R, editor. PLoS Comput Biol. 2020 Apr 16;16(4): e1007704.
3. Ware, Mark, and Michael Mabe. The STM report: An overview of scientific and scholarly journal publishing. 2015;
4. Grimshaw JM, Eccles MP, Lavis JN, Hill SJ, Squires JE. Knowledge translation of research findings. Implementation Sci. 2012 Dec;7(1):50.
5. Shoja MM, Walker TP, Carmichael SW. How to Find a Suitable Journal for Your Manuscript. In: Shoja M, Arynchyna A, Loukas M, D'Antoni AV, Buerger SM, Karl M, et al., editors. A Guide to the Scientific Career [Internet]. 1st ed. Wiley; 2019 [cited 2024 Apr 13]. p.389–402.Availablefrom: https://onlinelibrary.wiley.com/doi/10.1002/9781118907283.ch42
6. Hammad M. Criteria and Tips for Choosing Suitable Journal for Your Paper. 2023 [cited 2024 Apr 13]
7. Scopus. 2024; Available from: https://www.scopus.com/search/form.uri?display=basic#basic.
8. Web of Science. 2024;
9. Onwuegbuzie AJ, Mallette MH, Hwang E, Slate JR. Editorial: Evidence-based Guidelines for Avoiding Poor Readability in Manuscripts Submitted to Journals for Review for Publication. 2013;20(1):i–xi.
10. Cook DA. Twelve tips for getting your manuscript published. Medical Teacher. 2016 Jan 2;38(1):41–50.
11. Rosenfeld RM. How to review journal manuscripts. Otolaryngol--head neck surg. 2010 Apr;142(4):472–86.
12. Muka T, Glisic M, Milic J, Verhoog S, Bohlius J, Bramer W, et al. A 24-step guide on how to design, conduct, and successfully publish a systematic review and meta-analysis in medical research. Eur J Epidemiol. 2020 Jan;35(1):49–60.
13. Pickering C, Byrne J. The benefits of publishing systematic quantitative literature reviews for PhD candidates and other early-career researchers. Higher Education Research & Development. 2014 May 4;33(3):534–48.

Chapter 10

PATENTS

Guarding Innovation: Patenting Your Research Achievements.

10.1 Patent

The term "intellectual property rights" (IPR) refers to the legal protection of works of literature, art, inventions, designs, names, symbols, and images used in trade. Usually, these rights give the owner or author the only right to utilize their creation for a predetermined time. Trade secrets, industrial designs, trademarks, patents, and copyrights are all included. A patent is a type of intellectual property rights (IPR) that gives the owner exclusive rights to their innovation, usually for 20 years from the filing date and covered by the Indian Patent Act of 1970. The Food and Drug Administration (FDA) approves patents before they are granted by the Patent and Trademark Office (PTO). The Patent Act aims to balance protecting inventors' rights while promoting public interest and fostering economic growth, technological advancement, and technology transfer. Granting patents, fosters competition by preventing unauthorized copying or imitation of inventions, which motivates inventors to keep inventing (1). Three steps comprise the patent application process: filing, reviewing the application, and issuing the patent. During the patent prosecution phase, the PTO assesses the patent from a legal perspective; the claimed invention must be relevant to the patentable subject matter and be novel, valuable, and nonobvious. Processes, equipment, manufacturing techniques, compounds, and advancements over pre-existing versions of the goods above are all eligible for patent protection. However, patents are unavailable for abstract concepts or natural phenomena (2). Systems based on patents may encourage innovation, yet drug prices have reached all-time highs due to patent abuse. These rising costs have hampered the availability of essential pharmaceuticals (3).

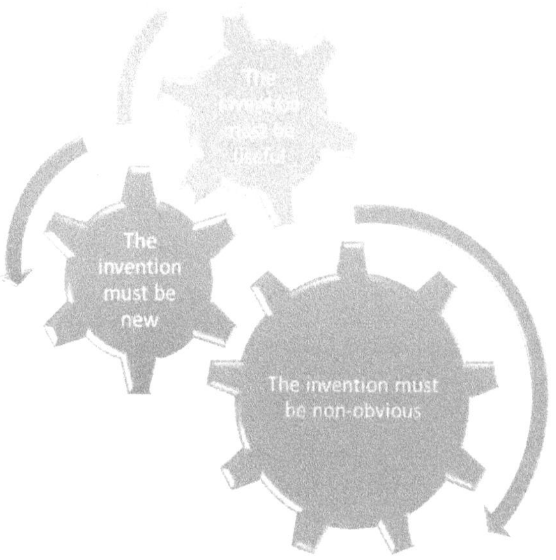

Image 10.1: Criteria for a patent.

10.2 Importance of patents

In the pharmaceutical domain, patents are essential because they promote investment, stimulate innovation, and guarantee patient access to medications. Key reasons that highlight their significance in the pharmaceutical sector are as follows:

a) **Incentivizing innovation**: Patents provide pharmaceutical companies exclusive rights to their inventions, including new drugs, formulations, and treatment methods. This exclusivity incentivizes companies to invest in costly research and development (R&D) efforts to discover and develop new medicines. Without the promise of patent protection, many companies would be less inclined to invest in the risky and expensive drug discovery.

b) **Promoting R&D investment:** The pharmaceutical sector invests heavily in research, and it takes a lot of money to bring a new drug from discovery to the market (4). By granting a period of market exclusivity, patents give businesses a way to recover the expenses of their R&D investments Because of their patents' exclusivity, businesses can charge more for their medications, which helps to pay for further research and development (5,6).

c) **Encouraging competition:** Besides giving the patent holder exclusive rights, patents promote competition once they expire. Other businesses will be able to manufacture generic versions of the medication once the patent term expires, which is usually 20 years from the date of application. This will increase competition and drive down prices. Patients gain from these since more reasonably priced medications are now available.

d) **Protecting intellectual property**: Patents protect pharmaceutical companies' intellectual property rights, preventing competitors from copying or exploiting their innovations without permission. This protection is essential for fostering innovation and ensuring companies are incentivised to invest in R&D.

e) **Facilitating collaboration:** Patents can be the foundation for cooperation and licensing contracts between academic institutions, pharmaceutical businesses, and research facilities. These agreements allow the sharing of information, funds, and technology, which promotes the creation of novel medications and treatments (7).

f) **Improving healthcare:** In the end, patents promote innovation, which advances public health. Patented inventions can produce novel medications and treatments that cure illnesses, lessen suffering, and enhance patients' quality of life all over the world (8).

10.3 Types of patents in the pharmaceutical domain

Patents are divided into 5 types

- Method of use
- Utility
- Design
- Process
- Product.

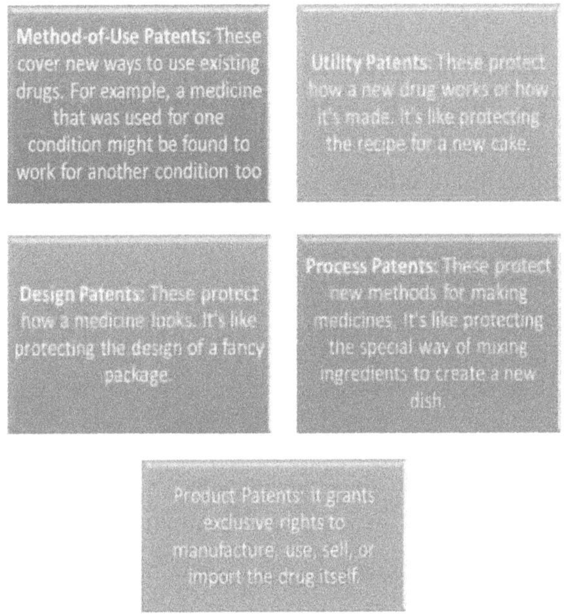

Fig no: 10.1 Types of patents (9).

10.4 How do you file patents?

Research and document your invention: Before filing a patent, thoroughly research your invention to ensure it is unique and not already patented by someone else. Document all details of your invention, including its composition, method of manufacture, and potential applications.

Conduct a patent search: Use online databases and resources to search for existing patents related to your invention. This step helps you determine if your invention is novel and non-obvious and the critical criteria for patentability. E.g. Google patent (10). The following documents are essential to file a patent registration application in India:

Patent Registration Application Form-1. Complete Specifications Form-2. In the absence of complete specifications, a provisional specification can be submitted.

Draft a patent application: Prepare a detailed patent application that describes the invention clearly and concisely. Include drawings, diagrams, or other visual aids to illustrate your invention's features and functionality.

Choose the correct type of patent: Decide whether your invention qualifies for a utility, design, or another type of patent based on its nature and characteristics. Utility patents are most common for new drugs, formulations, and manufacturing processes in the pharmaceutical domain. E.g. Design, Utility, Process, or Method of Use type of patent

File the patent application: Submit your application to the relevant patent office, such as the United States Patent and Trademark Office (USPTO) or the European Patent Office (EPO). Include the required forms, fees, and supporting documents with your application.

Wait for examination: After filing, your patent application will undergo examination by a patent examiner. The examiner will review your application to ensure it meets the criteria for patentability, including novelty, non-obviousness, and usefulness (11).

Respond to office actions: During the examination, the patent examiner may issue office actions requesting additional information or raising objections to your application. Respond promptly to address the examiner's concerns and provide clarification or amendments as needed.

Receive patent grant: If the patent office determines that your invention meets all requirements for patentability, they will grant you a patent. Once granted, your patent will provide you with exclusive rights to your invention for a specified period, typically 20 years from the filing date.

Maintain and enforce your patent: To maintain the validity of your patent and protect your exclusive rights from any possible infringers, you must pay maintenance fees.

Consider international protection: If you intend to commercialise your idea internationally, consider applying for foreign patent protection through regional or international patent systems, such as the Patent Cooperation Treaty (PCT). This enables you to obtain patent protection with a single application across several nations. The procedure for submitting a pharmaceutical patent application and safeguarding your discoveries against unapproved use or exploitation (12).

10.5 Controller general of patents, designs, and trademarks in India

- The Office of the Controller General of Patents, Designs & Trade Marks (CGPDTM) is in Mumbai.
- The Head Office of the Patent office is in Kolkata, and its Branch offices are in Chennai, New Delhi, and Mumbai.
- The Trade Marks registry is in Mumbai, and its Branches are in Kolkata, Chennai, Ahmedabad, and New Delhi.
- The Design Office is in Kolkata in the Patent Office.

- The Offices of The Patent Information System (PIS) and National Institute of Intellectual Property Management (NIIPM) are in Nagpur (13).

10.6 References

1. Chudasama, Dhaval, and Smit Patel. Importance of Intellectual Property Rights. Journal of Intellectual Property Rights Law. 2021;4(2):16–22.
2. Baruffaldi SH, Simeth M. Patents and knowledge diffusion: The effect of early disclosure. Research Policy. 2020 May;49(4):103927.
3. Jurek D. Patents, innovation, and market entry. Journal of Open Innovation: Technology, Market, and Complexity. 2024 Mar;10(1):100246.
4. How do pharmaceutical patents contribute to increased drug costs? Available from: https://pharmanewsintel.com/features/how-pharmaceutical-patents-contribute-to-increased-drug-costs
5. Kim J, Valentine K. The innovation consequences of mandatory patent disclosures. Journal of Accounting and Economics. 2021 Apr;71(2–3):101381.
6. Romasanta AKS, Van Der Sijde P, Van Muijlwijk-Koezen J. Innovation in pharmaceutical R&D: mapping the research landscape. Scientometrics. 2020 Dec;125(3):1801–32.
7. Why are the patents important? Available from: https://www.upcounsel.com/why-are-drug-patents-important
8. Resende Ferreira VV, Ricetto GC, Gaydeczka B, Granato AC, Pointer Malpass GR. Patents, what are they good for? Academic chemistry researcher's perceptions of patents and their importance. World Patent Information. 2022 Sep;70:102124.
9. Fredriksson M. India's Traditional Knowledge Digital Library and the Politics of Patent Classifications. Law Critique. 2023 Apr;34(1):1–19.
10. Choi JU, Lee CY. Do government-funded patents have higher quality than privately-funded patents? Economics of Innovation and New Technology. 2023 May 19;32(4):537–62.
11. Klincewicz K, Szumiał S. Successful patenting—not only how, but with whom: the importance of patent attorneys. Scientometrics. 2022 Sep;127(9):5111–37.

12. Kanwar S, Sperlich S. Innovation, productivity and intellectual property reform in an emerging market economy: evidence from India. Empir Econ. 2020 Aug;59(2):933–50.
13. Solanki, Nitesh. Review the organizational structure of the office of the controller general of patents, designs, trademarks, and geographical indications.

Rationale of the book

This book offers extensive and valuable advice for researchers starting with pharmaceutical studies and doctoral dissertation writing. The contributors provide precise, detailed instructions covering every phase of the research process, from choosing a topic to sharing findings, because they know the intricacies and difficulties that come with it. Essential topics covered in the book include writing a professional thesis, conducting literature reviews, planning experimental methods, and guaranteeing ethical human and animal research procedures. The book promises to provide researchers with the information and abilities required to succeed academically and professionally in the pharmaceutical sciences through helpful guidance, software tool recommendations, and communication techniques.

Summary of the book

This thorough manual is vital for researchers since it covers every pharmaceutical research and thesis composing stage. It starts with methods for choosing a study topic that is both possible and relevant. Key areas of exploration are identified by utilizing resources such as YouTube, LinkedIn, published papers, and reviews. The book leads users through creating a synopsis and offers precise, step-by-step guidance on successfully communicating your research. Essential phases of carrying out an exhaustive literature study are addressed, guaranteeing that you establish a firm basis by examining current material and pinpointing deficiencies. After that, the book moves on to planning and carrying out experiments, emphasising the significance of physicochemical characterisation, drug and excipient compatibility, and formulation development.

It emphasises using QbD principles to optimise and evaluate various dosage forms alongside in vitro studies. Practical aspects of conducting animal and human studies ethically and effectively are addressed, followed by guidance on writing a compelling thesis. The book underscores the significance of professional writing in achieving a doctoral certificate and provides tips for image preparation, crucial for thesis writing. It also discusses various statistical, drug design, and research writing software tools.

Finally, the guide prepares you for defending your thesis and offers advice on publishing and disseminating your findings to ensure your research reaches a broader audience. With its step-by-step approach and accessible language, this book is an invaluable companion for researchers embarking on pharmaceutical research and thesis writing across diverse fields.

Acknowledgements

The authors are grateful to Pristyn Research Solutions for providing the necessary facilities for book writing.

Conflict of interest:

The authors declare no conflict of interest

Final thoughts

The authors of this comprehensive guide express their final thoughts with a sense of fulfilment and hope that the book serves as an invaluable resource for researchers. They emphasize the guide's thorough coverage of the entire research process, from topic selection and literature review to experimental design and thesis writing. They aim to equip researchers with practical tools and clear strategies to navigate the complexities of pharmaceutical research, ultimately facilitating the achievement of academic and professional milestones. The authors aspire for this guide to be a trusted companion, fostering confidence and competence in researchers as they embark on their scientific endeavours.

Payal Jayendra Badole.

A Comprehensive Step-by-Step Guide for PhD Research Students" is an essential resource for navigating the complexities of doctoral research. From selecting a research topic to patenting your findings, this guide provides in-depth strategies and practical advice. It covers crucial aspects such as utilizing various tools and software, writing a compelling thesis, preparing a synopsis, and successfully defending your viva voce. This book is designed to equip PhD students with the knowledge and skills to excel in their research journey and achieve their academic goals. Whether you're just starting or nearing the end of your PhD, this guide will be your invaluable companion.

Swarupa Mohan Wanole

Authors biography

Pathan Azher Khan:

Pathan Azher, the CEO and founder of Pristyn Research Solutions, brings a wealth of experience to the table. With a strong foundation in scientific research and development, he has excelled in both the corporate and academic worlds. His expertise in clinical research and regulatory affairs ensures Pristyn Research Solutions delivers exceptional results.

Pathan's dedication extends beyond his own company. His involvement with various business and corporate organizations demonstrates his commitment to the industry's advancement. His experience working in academia and as a training and placement officer provides a unique perspective on the needs and aspirations of pharmaceutical and healthcare science professionals. This deep understanding fuels his passion for helping others navigate successful careers in these fields.

Pathan's impressive credentials include numerous international publications and patents. His extensive knowledge and industry recognition have earned him invitations as a Guest of Honor at prestigious pharmacy and medical colleges across India. Pathan's journey exemplifies the valuable bridge between academic pursuit and real-world industry application.

Further reading:

Grab your dream job in pharma: Interview questions and answers.